Shadow's Pride

Shadow's Pride

(BASED ON THE TRUE STORY OF AREION)

An Inspirational Account of
Courage, Determination and Love

Roland Stanzione and Gabriella Gafni

To order additional copies of this book, contact:
Xlibris Corporation
1-888-795-4274
www.Xlibris.com
Orders@Xlibris.com
57421

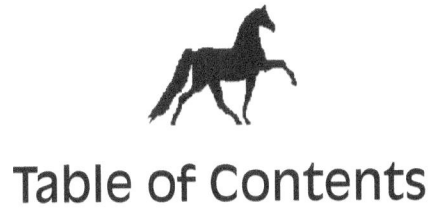

Table of Contents

Dedication 7

Acknowledgments 9

Prologue 11

Introduction 13

Chapter 1: The Legend of Areion 15

Chapter 2: Roland's Song 17

Chapter 3: The World Through My Eyes 20

Chapter 4: Two Against The World 25

Chapter 5: On The Road Again 31

Chapter 6: Joyful Engagements 36

Chapter 7: In and Out of Darkness 39

Chapter 8: Destiny's Two Faces 43

Chapter 9: Treading On Uncertain Ground 47

Chapter 10: Living In The Moment 52

Chapter 11: My Four-Leaved Clover 57

Chapter 12: Life's Tests 59

Chapter 13: To Sleep, Perchance To Dream 63

Chapter 14: A Synchronized Reverie 68

Chapter 15: At Rainbow's End 79

Chapter 16: I Am Spirit 85

Chapter 17: Commemoration 87

Chapter 18: Epilogue 89

Dedication

(To Areion, whose spirit slipped the bounds of earth on
October 27, 2006, forever my Brother).

Areion, you lived a life which no being should have to endure, filled with old wounds, injuries and pain. In addition to health problems, you were confronted with prejudice and discrimination. In my eyes, you were a light in the darkness.

I gave everything of myself and within my power to show you how much I cared. I wanted to teach you how to trust and to love, attributes which reflected in your eyes. You were strong and stalwart, carrying me in times of weakness and uncertainty. Despite every inflicted wrongdoing and misconception, you grazed contentedly, ever seeking the promise of a new dawn. When walking side by side in green grass and clover and riding together, we were immune to life's tribulations, emboldened by our loving friendship.

I never thought about the day when we would not be together. By your display of strength, courage, and love of life, you inspired me. Your belief in me provided purpose in the sometimes aimlessness of existence. Through your example, I learned many lessons, and I am grateful to God that you came into my life, albeit much too briefly. The night your heart stopped beating, I not only lost my best friend, but my heart's core. I knelt beside your warm body as autumnal darkness and rain fell upon us. One year later, when I revisited the site, the sky again sent cascades of tears, representing our parting and how much we miss one another; but, like always, you then showed me the sun and enlivened in me the need to realize the dressage dreams we shared. In times of grief, I am ever reminded of your courage, and my only solace is that you and I will meet again at Heaven's Gate and run together freely. Until then, God will keep you in safe pastures and your hoof prints will remain in my heart.

"You were my strength when I was weak,
You were my voice when I couldn't speak,
You were my eyes when I couldn't see,
You saw the best there was in me.
Lifted me up when I couldn't reach,
You gave me faith 'cause you believed.
I'm everything I am
Because you loved me."

Lyrics by Diane Warren and produced by David Foster for the film *Up Close & Personal*, sung by Céline Dion

Acknowledgments

This book is a tribute not only to my best friend, Areion, but also to those who touched our lives and sustained us on our journey together. From the bottom of my heart, I extend profound thanks to the following outstanding individuals:

Anne and Connie Stanzione, my family, for their love and support.

Dr. Benson Martin of the University of Pennsylvania Veterinary School, New Bolton Center, for his extraordinary display of expertise, competence and empathy.

Dr. Patty Hogan of the New Jersey Equine Clinic, for her unparalleled care and insight, and for giving Areion a lease on life, I will always be grateful.

Dr. Dean Richardson of the University of Pennsylvania Veterinary School, New Bolton Center, for his vast, inspirational contributions to the field and the creation of the Barbaro Research Fund, an initiative dedicated to laminitis research and other equine health and safety issues.

Dr. Tiffany Marr of The Mid-Atlantic Equine Medical Center and Erica, her technical assistant, for their graciousness and guidance in one of the most trying hours of my life.

Mr. Scott Previte, farrier, for his extensive talents and professionalism, and for giving his all to Areion.

Michael and Elizabeth-Perry Mebler and Staff of High Brass Farm Equine Rehabilitation Center for their indefatigable efforts in Areion's treatment and care.

Dominique, Gerry, and Steve Cassavetis, for their inspiration and steadfast friendship.

Paul Placenti, for his encouragement, friendship, and zealous promotion of this work.

Ms. Susan Villani, Areion's kind, caring rehab walker.

Maggie McGuire and Renegate of Performance Farm in Whitehouse, NJ, for giving me the opportunity to ride again with a Grand Prix-level horse.

Mr. Michael Schlueter, cover-designer, for his masterful artistry.

Ms. Rachel DeRagon, artist, for her beautiful rendering of the dream sequence painting.

Lorraine Patricia Photography, for displaying superior professionalism and expertise.

Prologue

Every life finds meaning in another when worlds converge. A leap of faith emanates from the heart, where bonds are forged. Such a connection took place with my equine friend, Areion, from the moment I beheld him. Everything in his manner, stance and spirit spoke to the fact that he yearned to belong, that he needed me. Little did we know, at the outset, that I would come to rely on his strength.

When I first met Areion, he viewed human beings with suspicion and fear. He reared up, reacting to past experiences of loneliness and poor treatment. His owner had abandoned him. Without a name or registration papers, he searched for an identity, a home. Somehow, he knew that his very life was at stake. A series of health issues (specifically, a fracture which shattered his right knee, navicular degeneration in both feet, and laminitis) consigned him to an awful fate. Shipped from the Midwest to central New Jersey, he was to be sold at auction and, most likely, sent to slaughter.

Notwithstanding his underdog status, Areion clung to his last chance with every fiber. He emerged into the arena of his new barn, prepared for scrutiny and evaluation, with stoic pride and self-awareness, intent on impressing the barn owner. Inconspicuously, I watched. Areion's demeanor revealed his inner spirit, begging for a rescue, defying his underlying vulnerability. Such pristine innocence captivated me and, had I dismissed the opportunity of meeting such a creature, I would have denied my very Self. In the performance of a lifetime, fighting against all odds, Areion pranced, jumped, and executed lead-changes gracefully. His huge brown eyes, encapsulating his soul's dignity, seemed to cast off the shadow of his doleful past. When I approached and spoke to him, we formed an instantaneous, indelible attachment. Soon, Areion became my "Shadow's Pride."

Our lives joined. Each of us intrinsically understood the supreme importance of character, empathy and understanding when juxtaposed with outer appearance and calculable value. Called an "appendix" (i.e., part quarter horse, half thoroughbred, with salient characteristics of the latter, due to his level of speed and grace), Areion possessed the shining inner qualities of a champion, longing for recognition based upon who he was, rather than on his monetary worth. Areion's life was a testament to the far-reaching power of unconditional love and desire to reach beyond limitations to be his best. For me, his exemplary life served as a metaphor for true courage.

In the following pages, I offer his story, alternating Areion's perspective with my own. In a fact-based account, tinged with some dramatic elements, I wish to demonstrate the iniquities of an industry which emphasizes monetary value and gain over individual attributes. In so doing, I hope to give Areion a voice, as well as to inspire others who stand on the periphery of society: the disenfranchised, the physically challenged, and all of those who need to find beauty in the journey, not simply in the destination.

Introduction

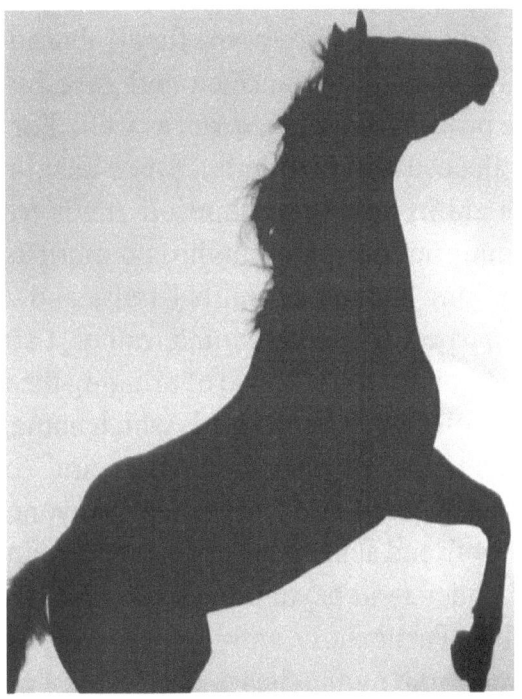

My journey toward the completion of this narrative was not easy. I was constantly weighed down by doubt and derision, told that I have "axes to grind" and "bridges to burn." These comments only served to overlook my earnest intentions. Of course, I was deeply hurt by the manner in which Areion was treated—particularly in his last days; naturally, I was—and ever remain—indignant about the way horses who are not considered "champions" are often destined for slaughter because of what humans deem to be their "imperfections;" and I am pained by the recollection of how barn owners turned Areion away because of his condition, viewing him as property to be bought, sold, nurtured as a champion or discarded. I take issue with the fact that these conditions are placed upon horses' survival. We have lawsuits to redress discrimination in the human sphere; but upon whom can our equine friends rely?—The very humans who judge them. Endowed with the ability to reason, we, as humans, have the responsibility to voice concerns about how animals are treated and their intrinsic worth.

In my view, Areion was a prototype for all abused and neglected creatures. I saw beneath the surface and gave him a chance at survival. In the process, *he rescued me*, as well. For these reasons, I take creative license and give him a voice as co-narrator of his story. Areion's ability to express himself stems from his name's connection to anthropomorphic (an·thro·po·mor·fic) gods—those capable of assuming human or animal traits and attributes. Of course, I don't purport to read his mind; rather, I attempt to place myself in his position for the purpose of bringing the reader into our world. Since Areion cannot form words which humans understand, his communication most often occurs "in the spirit" (or the depths of his being—a place beyond physical matter). Anyone who has a pet family member or friend acknowledges in these creatures the ability to "speak" and understand beyond the spoken word as we humans conceive it to be. Particularly with horses, a profundity of spirit emanates, pervades the human heart, and forms a connection.

Areion was a real horse with a very real story, narrated here factually and authentically. My greatest apprehension was fictionalizing issues which I consider to be intensely personal and dear; but, by interlacing creative elements with actual happenings, I hope to adorn my tribute with the poignancy which a loving, grateful heart best can render.

Chapter 1

The Legend of Areion
(Areion's Narrative)

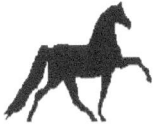

I live in my mind, where I run with the wind. In imagination's realm, no barriers exist. Judgment, prejudice and misconception are subsumed in my power. I run freely, unfettered by time and circumstance. As my name connotes, I am an immortal horse, child of the Sea and Earth, son of Poseidon and Demeter, metamorphosed as stallion and mare, to engender my invincible form.[1] Descending from the lineage of gods, I have been heralded by the Poet as the swiftest of steeds.[2] Speaking in praise of me, he wrote: "[In a chariot race, there] is none who could sprint to make it up, nor close you, nor pass you, not if the man behind you were driving the great Areion . . . ."[3] In glorious hours, I rode with mighty Heracles and, then, was entrusted to Adrestos, whose life I saved at Thebes. Were it not for me, he would have perished, as all the others.[4] I am a rescuer of hearts, a patron of humanity, wanting nothing, giving

---

[1] According to Greek mythology, Areion was born to Poseidon, God of the Sea, and Demeter, Goddess of Agriculture. To escape Poseidon's pursuit, Demeter transformed into Erinys, a mare. The Sea God, in turn, became a stallion, to engender Areion and a daughter, whose identity, to date, remains unknown. Though initially wrathful, Demeter/Erynis conceded acceptance.

[2] Areion makes reference to Homer, legendary poet of ancient Greece, born ca. 8th century, B.C.E.

[3] Homer, Iliad 23.346.

[4] Aeschylus' play (467 B.C.), *Seven Against Thebes*, depicts the devastating battle of two brothers who vie for ascension to the throne of their father, Oedipus, and kill each other in single combat. Their armies perish as well, save for Adrestos, who was rescued by Areion.

much, and prancing through my world with mane afire, black as night. My eyes are receptacles and transmitters of love, radiating joy in existence.

Were my lauded days so long ago? When will I rescue again? Oh, to dance in the splendid, graceful harmony of dressage, where horses' and riders' hearts beat in tandem, to float on air like a gallant ballet performer, testimony to the practices of my ancestors, the ancient Greeks, and their progeny, the Lipizzaner stallions of Vienna and, later, of Italy and Austria! The precision in movement, the touch of my comrade's hand, the teamwork: it all lies within my capacity!

A sudden clap of thunder resounds around me. I wince and cower. I lower my foot to the ground, toe first. A shocking, deeply painful reality pervades my being. Physical anguish envelopes me, as I involuntarily close my eyes. Slowly, I gaze up above me. I am alone, in my stable, my foot smarting. The star-filled sky is obscured to my vision. I feel solitude, but not fear. I realize that this is not all that I am or can be. I am comprised of the stuff of legend and, at once, the cold present; but I am so much more.

"Areion, live!" I cry out. "So much awaits!" The darkness listens and seems to beckon my patience. I hearken more to hear my friend, the wind, calling: "Silence, wait, your knight will come!"

Chapter 2

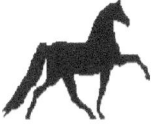

Roland's Song[5]
(Roland's Narrative)

Count Roland am I, in time's lore sketched,
In history praised, eternally etched.
Through Roncesvaux[6] I blithely ride,
With liege Olivier[7] at my side.
In service of Great Charlemagne,
I travel forth on foes' terrain
To preserve the honor of my friends,
And vanquish wrathful Saracens.
I sally on, with Veillantif,[8]
Stout of heart, of firm belief.
With Durindana[9] clasped in hand,
I vow to conquer land for land,
Shielding comrades from shame and harm.
Hark! I hear a strange alarm!

I rise from my bed with a start, standing almost upright. Holding the side of my head, I jump back and strike out at my alarm clock, as though I were facing mortal combat. The noise ceases.

---

[5] The opening salvo of Chapter 2 parodies "The Song of Roland," the earliest in the French tradition of "chansons de geste" ("songs of heroic deeds"). The epic poem, dating from the late eleventh to early twelfth centuries, depicts the valiant deeds of Count Roland, nephew of Charlemagne, King of the Franks, in his battle against the Saracens (777-778 A.D.).

[6] Roncesvaux: Territory of the Saracens, formerly Basques.

[7] Olivier: Roland's trusted friend.

[8] Veillantif: Roland's horse.

[9] Durindana: Roland's sword.

"What just happened?" I ask myself aloud. I feel as if I have emerged from a time-tunnel. I cup my face in my hands and, then, slowly allow my eyes to search the familiar space of my room. The only vestiges of my armor are a football helmet, a set of old shoulder pads, and riding boots. My sword, Durindana, has transformed into tricep bars and handles. For a moment, a fleeting thought occurs: I have abandoned King Charlemagne. Then, smiling to myself, I transition easily into the present. I glance quickly at my horse calendar, and a sense of anticipation envelopes me. I realize that, today, I will do something which I have not undertaken since college.

Courtesy of my sister, Connie, I will leave for Washington Stables[10] for the first in a series of Western riding lessons. We plan to travel together in one truck and, then, divide into groups of four. I am filled with excitement, coupled with a hint of anxiety. I have not experienced the freedom and beauty of riding horses in over twenty years, but my connection to those magnificent animals summons me forth.

Washington Stables is a farm, of sorts, an open field with a trail and an old barn, scarcely off of a main street. During the lessons, my group rides through trails, then stops, forms a circle and engages in balance-training exercises, consisting of controlled limb movements. Then, the group gallops in a straight line, trying to remain as one cohesive unit. Such training conduces to speed, control and straightness. Then, one-by-one, each of us independently trots, gallops, comes to a complete stop, and proceeds to the trail's end. Next, we perform turning drills, which simulate relay races. Without the instructor's guidance, the two groups fan out in different directions with the goal of returning to the original assemblage. I can only imagine what feats my historic counterpart, Count Roland of my dream, accomplished in his time!

The euphoria and delight I feel when performing such tasks hardly can be expressed. The sheer power of the horses takes my breath away.

---

[10]   At the time of this writing the, Washington Stables no longer exists.

I am awed by the animals' physical and spiritual grandeur. Never have I witnessed such heart in living beings. My aptitude develops quickly, as the instructor indicates. Her encouragement bolsters me to such a degree that, by the fourth lesson, I purchase my own saddle, declaring that which I have been given to be "not good enough." At this moment, I openly acknowledge that I want my own horse. Much akin to Charlemagne's nephew, I seek new opportunities, challenges, and connections to and with horses. I finish my time at Washington Stables, and set out for Silver Saddle Farms in Readington, New Jersey, where the owner's son, Dave Kraft, coaxes me to begin English-style riding lessons. These differ considerably from Western riding lessons in technique and verbal expressions for the movements. I also receive positive reinforcement about dressage training, a challenging, graceful discipline, similar to dancing with horses. Oh, to establish such a partnership, a symbiosis of hearts!

Silver Saddle's staff trainer, Jennifer, and I discuss free-style dressage. She works with and sells school horses. Sale is the most important aspect of the equestrian "business." Windman, a "paint horse" (i.e. a combination of white and other equine colors), comes to my attention. A taciturn young horse, his carriage reveals self-consciousness and inexperience. As he approaches me, Windman lowers and thrusts his head forward. The white, grey and brown steed studies me with mismatched eyes of brown and blue. The embodiment of beauty, he does not speak to me. We are both amateurs, with nothing to declare or offer to one another. Yet, my yearning to commence life as an equestrian prompts me to purchase him for $7,500. Jennifer, who naturally endorses the sale, knows full well that Windman and I, the Uninitiated, are both "painted"—green. For such reason, my relationship with Windman lasts for about a week to ten days, after which period my life truly begins, as I witness a vehicle arrive at Silver Saddle Farms, hailing from the Midwest.

Chapter 3

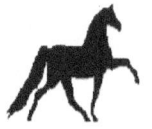

The World Through My Eyes
(Areion's Narrative)

*D*awn breaks, and a canopy of solitude envelopes me. Though I cannot view the sky, I sense that freedom dwells there. Perhaps, I can look to the sun for answers. When I raise my head upward, I feel that new and hopeful possibilities await. Can this be true for a so-called "hack horse,"[11] unrecognized, unaccustomed to human kindness? I know who I am, I have a name. Maybe, today, someone will take notice and I can be free.

My stall door opens and a gruff voice calls out: "Come on, boy!" I am ushered quickly into a huge trailer, hauled forth like property. According to humankind's definition I am, merely, "chattel," to be bought and sold, evaluated for monetary worth, owned for profit, not prized for the contents of my soul. I have an identifiable heart and spirit, yearning to live, to reach the full breath of my potential, to give to people and to the world; but no one knows. Dollar signs often cloud human vision and compassion. Still, I cling to hope.

Although human language is foreign to me, I understand general meanings, which I mentally process and translate through observation. On this particular day, I sense that I will travel from my stall in Oklahoma to an auction in Cranbury, New Jersey, where owners buy creatures like me for trail riding. Instantly, terror seizes me. What if the evaluation goes badly and the owners do not like me? I will go to slaughter! As the pain in my left foot reminds me, I am in peril. To make matters worse, my right knee hurts from an old fracture which I sustained as a cutting horse.[12] To this day,

---

[11] Hack horses are used for trail riding.

[12] The sport requires horses to make sharp turns and short stops.

bone fragments remain in my right knee, but no one has bothered to have me vetted.

I wish that I had someone to watch over me, as the lady sings in the song I heard from my stall one night.[13] Sometimes, I hear music as it floats on the air in range of my hearing; but no one ever sings to me or even speaks kindly in my direction. I suppose that, in my owners' eyes, I am not important. Such impressions do not matter, however, for I possess the greatest resource: my pride, of which no being or circumstance can rob me! "I resolve to be at my best. I will show them!" I declare loudly to myself.

Suddenly, I hear a loud command: "Be still, boy!" I realize that I must have neighed aloud. When one lives alone as much as I do, inner conversations become second nature. The journey seems endless, and I fight a fever welling up in my body. I have a plan, a life-saving scheme which, I only hope, will catch someone's attention.

As I disembark from the trailer, spent of energy, beset with pain, I lift my head to the sun and sky. "At last, you are visible! Shine down and lend me support." Rays of light beam an affirmative reply. The auctioneers walk, trot and run with me for the bidding public. Never have I felt so compelled to challenge myself. Despite my ailments, I accomplish my tasks with elegance and dignity. I am, after all, of noble heritage. A woman in the crowd observes me with interest and begins her bid. This is it! I rejoice in my success, as I hear the auctioneer exclaim: "Sold to the lady in blue!" Betty Kraft steps forward and beckons me: "There is my fine trail horse!" Her demeanor is flavored with good humor. I follow, grateful to be given a chance.

---

[13] A reference to the song "Someone to Watch Over Me," composed by George Gershwin, with lyrics by Ira Gershwin from the musical *Oh, Kay!* (1926), where Getrude Lawrence introduced it. Since the song's debut, it has been recorded by numerous artists and is a jazz standard and key work in the Great American Songbook.

Betty has her own trailer, a cut above that to which I have been accustomed, but the trip wreaks havoc upon my knee and foot. The bumpy roads make me weary, and the pain in my left foot is indescribable. Through the entire journey, I feel fortunate just to be alive, to be given safe shelter.

Nightfall arrives once more. Somehow, time's transition occurs in spite of me. I am glad to rest, hardly observing my new surroundings, a farm called "The Silver Saddle." I sleep without dreaming, and awaken to a flurry of activity. Eight to ten trail horses, tied under trees, clamor a short distance from my stall. Quite against their will, they wait to take outsiders for rides through the woods. Most of the riders are inept, and the horses sense their incompetence. Betty does not care how they feel, as her sights remain on the hourly fee. She compels the horses to ride, despite their protestations. Does she not understand? At all cost, I must avoid a similar fate. Perhaps, I will be discovered and rescued. Now is my chance. When the trainer, Jane, takes me to the arena for exercise today, I will exert my strength and pride for all the onlookers.

The fenced outdoor arena lies past an old barn, where Betty has her office. Covered with stone dust and sand, the place looks barren, devoid of warmth. Horse jumps (brown wooden poles between stands), three inches in width, populate the grounds. To the far right, I see pasture fields in deplorable condition. In a grassy area nearby, vet tests are performed in a round pen. How I wish that a doctor would examine my foot and knee! The pony pen below the arena captures my attention. Maybe, later, I can befriend my fellow equines! Thoughts flood my mind, in an attempt to stave off fear and uncertainty. Then, I collect myself and prepare for my ride with Jane.

I display eagerness when Jane comes for me. She is kind and comforting, and I feel lithe in her presence. Riding me first indoors, she then rounds the outdoor arena, so that Betty can view my jumping, trotting, and running prowess. Despite my intense pain, I perform every task, including two-foot jumps. I call forth every ounce of grace, strength and wit, which Jane recognizes. She commends me by caressing my neck. "Pain, you are nothing to me!" I scoff at my distress. "I am Areion, the Conqueror!" A low sound emanates from my throat. As I rear slightly, Jane asks me to be calm. Clearly, she is impressed.

Suddenly, a man walks toward the outdoor arena from the parking lot. For some reason, my heart skips a beat. He looks at me keenly and walks over to Betty, who now stands in the outdoor arena, watching me. From what I can detect, Betty explains that she has just purchased me. Gazing at me admiringly, the man appears gentle, of strong build, his eyes gleaming with integrity and earnestness. "I want to belong," I whisper. As if he hears me, the man approaches and Betty addresses him as "Roland." He comes out of time, like me! I exclaim to myself. Anticipation overtakes me, while I remain in performance mode. Dare I imagine that my knight has arrived?

"He is elegant and has a mind about him," Roland affirms. "If you will not tender a refund, can I make a fair trade of Windman?"

"Why do you want to do that? Windman is a good horse. A deal is a deal." Betty's look is a little mischievous. Money-making prospects are, always, inviting.

"Like me, Windman is inexperienced. I believe that I can have a greater connection with that horse."

I see The Gallant One gesturing toward me! What does it all mean? Oh, Fate, please be kind! Is my enthusiasm not evident? Where will life carry me now? My mind whirls with an admixture of excitement and trepidation. Roland approaches and, again, my heart plays strange music. Suddenly, I feel as though I wish to dance. My feet sway beneath me, but I maintain composure. As Roland takes my lead line and strokes me, I am instantly at peace.

Tonight, I rest awake, thinking of what first light will bring. Perhaps, Roland and I will be a team! The morning sunshine tells me that, soon, I will have to be vetted. "I will put him on a lunge line," the vet declares. "The clockwise and counterclockwise motions will reveal any deformities."

"A full vet exam would be best," Roland observes, revealing his immediate devotion.

"No, the exam is good enough for a horse like this." Betty's dismissive tone negates all hope of a complete checkup.

"Something is wrong with his left shoulder. He limps, due to an over-extension of the right leg. He is coming up short," the vet states flatly.

"Roland, you should not buy that horse," Dave, Betty's son, mutters to my hero. "There is something wrong with him."

"I see something special in him. I consider him, not his value as a show horse, as truly wonderful. Things are not always as they seem, and he has a lot beneath the surface. I can bond with him and deal with any problems which may arise." Roland, I sense that you see the world through my eyes." I nicker gently. My knight supposes that I am, simply, saying 'hello,' but my greeting holds infinite gratitude.

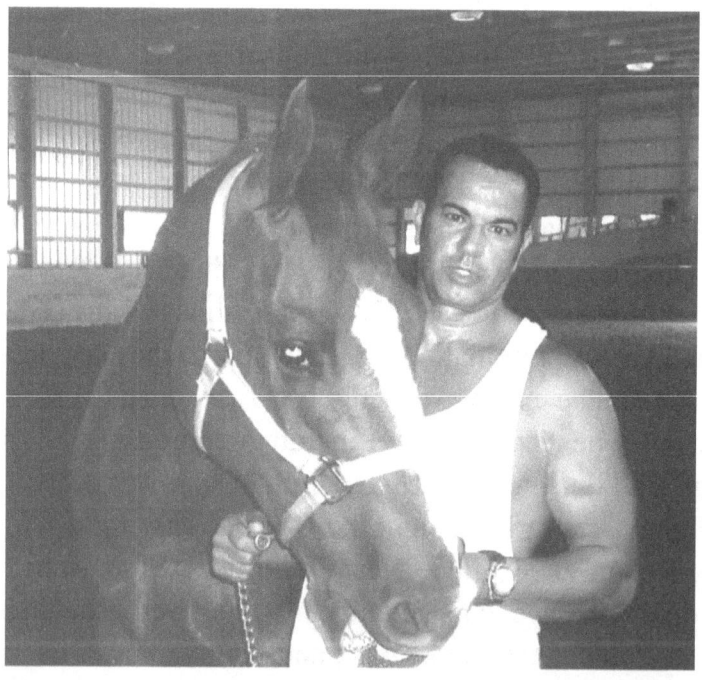

Chapter 4

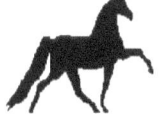

Two Against The World
(Roland's Narrative)

*I*nstantly, I recognize the horse's integrity and desire to please. He seems to speak to me in his spirit, asking for support. Betty hands him over without a paper trail, unregistered. I feel as though I have adopted a refugee, bereft of a home. "I will take care of you," I murmur softly to my new friend, whose soulful eyes seem to meet mine. I request a comfortable stall for him. At first, the horse shies away a bit, mistrustful of humans but, gradually, he warms up to me and we develop a strong emotional bond.

I set about researching a name for my noble waif, who deserves identification befitting his dignity. Greek mythology seems like a good place to begin, given its references to valiant horses. I believe in this creature, and am ready to give his life meaning, to share a dream of dancing in a beginner's dressage show, winning as a team. "Areion, immortal horse!" I call aloud to him one day. He nods in assent, as if in acknowledgment of a name he has heard before. Within a week, I give Areion his show name, "Shadow's Pride," so conferred for the cloud over his past and in homage to his ever-present sense of self.

The onset of Areion's one-hundred-five-degree shipping fever mars the joy of our newfound partnership. Areion looks piqued, perspires profusely, and is laden with fatigue. Filled with worry and empathy, I immediately request a visit from the Silver Saddle's veterinarian, Dr. Geoff Brant, who prescribes antibiotics and gives Areion an injection. One week elapses before my friend begins to feel like himself again. My daily visits and gifts of carrots and apples serve to keep his head up, but he still demonstrates profound weakness. I remain stoic, ready to face whatever comes.

As he begins to return to health, Areion grazes and tries to enjoy his surroundings, but finds the trail horses' ruckus distracting. On one occasion, when I approach the gate for a visit, I sense the horses running toward me. I am unafraid, but Areion believes that they are charging, and rears up against them as though he were battling for my life. The horses scatter, running in every direction. Not only am I amused but, also, convinced of Areion's complete devotion and our unshakable connection.

Life continues as usual until, in our third month together, Areion's limp worsens. Dr. Brant comes for a visit and renders a very cursory, general diagnosis, after which x-rays are taken. Dr. Brant is a man of few words, hording knowledge. His loyalty appears to be directed toward the Silver Saddle alone. His subsequent silence regarding the outcome of Areion's x-rays confirms my observations. Persistent calls to his office (over the course of what seems to be endless time) do not prompt a response, and my frustration grows daily.

Recognizing that my friend receives second-hand treatment, I try to contain my displeasure, as my anguish and worry increase with each passing moment. I feel the blood rise to my head, as I unsuccessfully attempt to determine Dr. Brant's whereabouts. Clearly, Areion suffers from a condition which must be addressed, but here we remain, in obscurity, deprived of crucial facts. I look over my shoulder to see Dave, Betty's son, stepping into the arena, as Areion's exam ends. Has Dave concealed something? What does Betty know? Perhaps, without my knowledge, Dr. Brant clandestinely gave the x-ray reports to them. Unjust practices in the equestrian realm brand Areion as 'a nobody;' but he means so much more to me. We are two against the world. As I spend several moments in deep reflection, the first stanza of an apt Emily Dickinson verse comes to mind, entitled "I'm Nobody! Who Are You?"[14]

---

[14] Emily Dickinson (1830-1886), American poet, known for her unique rhyming style and punctuation.

> I'm nobody! Who are you?
> Are you nobody, too?
> Then there's a pair of us—don't tell!
> They'd banish us, you know.

Banishment is not an option, as long as I have strength within me, I affirm silently in thought. I am startled from contemplation by a tap on the shoulder. Dave approaches me and I declare, in one breath: "If no one else will care for Areion, I must take swift, concerted action on my own." I quickly depart to make an urgent phone call.

Dr. Hans Nettherz[15], a U.S. Olympic-team veterinarian, has an office in Oldwick, New Jersey, just twenty minutes from the Silver Saddle. I prepare to take Areion there and explain my plans to him. Ever compliant, my friend nods consent. When we arrive, the doctor instructs the tech to trot Areion, commenting that he is a bit "out of shape." I take the doctor's observation to be a comparison to his customary Olympian equine patients. Dr. Nettherz and his staff then perform a nerve block to determine the source of Areion's pain. After being trotted with and without the block, the existence of a problem clearly surfaces, and x-rays are taken. My heart descends into my stomach when the doctor diagnoses Areion with navicular disease.[16]

---

[15] Dr. Nettherz's name is taken from two German words, *nett* and H*erz* which, in combination, mean "Nice Heart," reflecting his gracious demeanor. The original veterinarian's identity is withheld in deference to his privacy.

[16] Navicular disease, more properly termed "navicular syndrome," is inflammation or degeneration of the navicular bone (one of the tarsal bones located on the medial side of the foot). Symptoms of the condition proceed from a protrusion of the foot, caused by a lack of proper calcification of the three cuneiforms (i.e., medial, intermediate, and lateral) which compose the bone. The foot extension places stress on two tendons and the ligament alongside which, in turn, allow a so-called 'extra navicular bone' or bump to develop which strains the tendons and causes pain in movement (i.e., increased activity). In extreme cases, denerving surgery is performed.

Areion seems to catch my glance and observes my sorrow. He is stalwart, waiting for answers, as well. His eyes speak the words, "don't worry, Roland. We will get through this together." In an effort to avoid immediate surgery, Dr. Nettherz suggests shockwave therapy. Ultimately, contrary to our every hope, the procedure proves to be unsuccessful. Downcast and without recourse, I still do not give up hope. I wonder how we have come to this point, how everyone around us may know things about which I, Areion's guardian, am unfamiliar. Thus far, no one has offered any enlightenment. I head home and come to the barn early the next day, taking a day off from work. Betty offers to trailer us to the University of Pennsylvania Veterinarian School in New Bolton, where Dr. Benson Martin has his practice. She has done this a number of times for clients. Areion receives top-notch attention at New Bolton, irrespective of his underdog status (i.e. as an equine outside the high end echelon of equestrian show and race horses). Twenty competent, knowledgeable students surround and trot him, making him turn in a circle. Dr. Martin observes that he is lame. He performs a nerve block, jogs Areion again, and takes another series of x-rays. I watch nervously, as digital photos appear on the computer screen. The room is, roughly, the size of a two-car garage. Impressed and overwhelmed at once, I await the doctor's evaluation.

"Dr. Martin, what have you found?" I inquire anxiously. The doctor's distress is visible. "Areion has navicular disease," he states outright, his voice steady and kind. Your options are either special shoes or surgery. I can suggest a farrier in New Bolton."

"That's much too far, Doctor. I will find one closer to Areion's barn, the Silver Saddle," I affirm.

The doctor is troubled that a horse could be sold in such a condition.

Within the next few days, Areion and I go to a farrier, who constructs an aluminum shoe with a two-degree lift, appearing light and comfortable. However, even this proactive measure does not seem to have any positive effect on my friend, who continues to show a profound limp. His lack of progress causes me many sleepless nights, as I ponder my next step. When I visit Areion after work the next evening, I assure him that we will conquer the situation, as a team. Areion responds with gratitude for my carrots, bestowed generously during our conversation. I never feel as if I am speaking in vain when he is around. Our understanding of each other is implicit, as we are brothers, both in need of each other.

My next course of action takes place with Dr. Greg Samuels, a surgeon in Oldwick. He orders the digital x-rays from New Bolton and takes a new series, as well.

"Are there any options besides surgery? Will Areion always have pain? Am I going to lose him?" I inquire, barely able to breathe.

The doctor hesitates. "I am not in favor of euthanizing a young ten-year-old horse when I can treat him with surgery."

Reluctantly, but with resignation, I assent and ask whether the denerving procedure would be inhumane.

"Only part of the nerve will be taken from the left foot." Dr. Samuels tries to sound reassuring. "Areion will have to be on stall rest for six to eight weeks, without strenuous activity."

"You can count on us to follow your advice, Dr. Samuels." I muster every ounce of inner strength to appear optimistic.

While Areion is in the hospital, I decide to take lessons with the Silver Saddle school horses. As I step out into the mud one day, my right foot becomes stuck in a hole and my boot pulls straight off. I think nothing of the incident, until I have pain when I walk on my right foot. Perhaps, it is a dismount fracture, I muse to myself. Later, however, a doctor's visit reveals that I must have a cast. As the day advances, I only can think of Areion, however, and rush to his side to take him home. As I slowly amble into the hospital, my hero emerges with a huge wrap on his left foot. We are veritable foils of one another, quite an amusing duo. Everyone smiles and jokes, while I whisper to Areion, remembering the Dickinson poem: "Now, there is the pair of us—and I do not care that the world banishes us, for our dream lives and a new tomorrow awaits!"

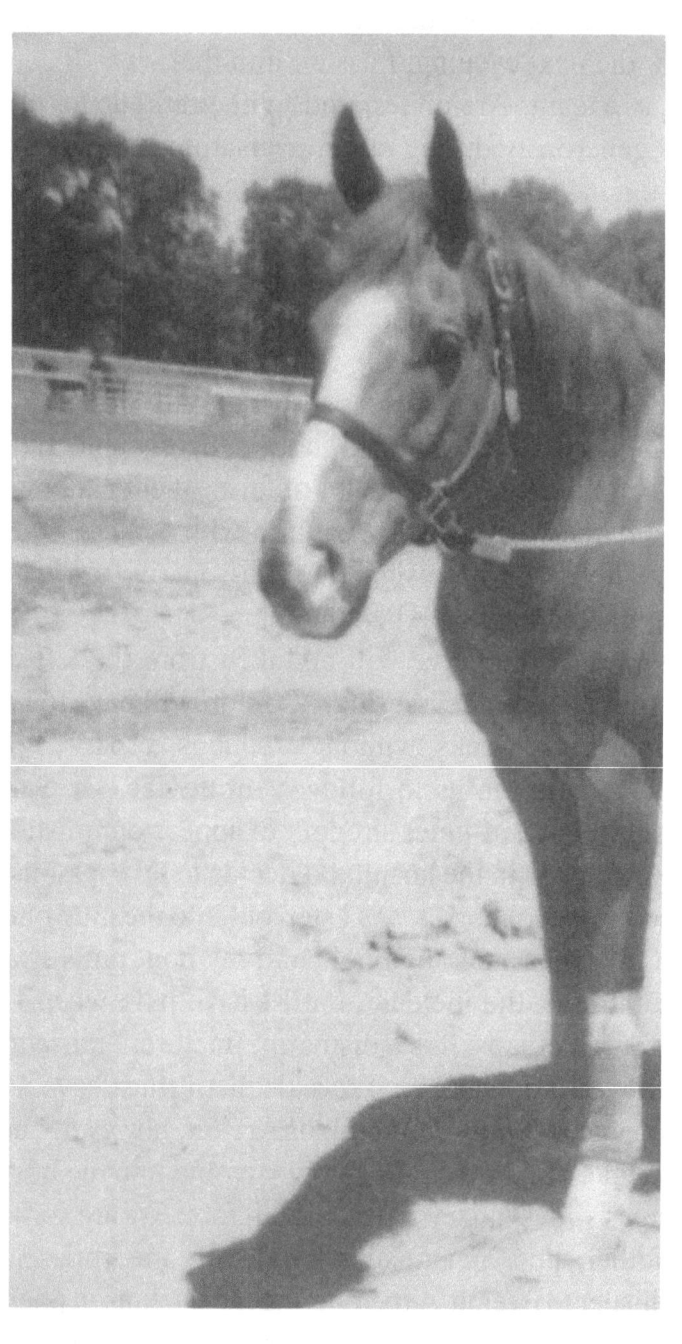

Chapter 5

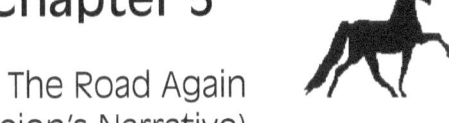

On The Road Again
(Areion's Narrative)

*a*fter surgery, I await my knight's rescue and my departure for home. I miss my friends, especially Dominique Cassavetis, a strong, talented young dressage rider, who always comes to check on me, her Mom, Gerry, and their elderly mustang, Nacho, who fears every man, except for Roland. My knight bestows security and friendship in the form of carrots. My old comrade has had a troubled past. Apparently, an inhumane human tied a wire around his tongue, leaving scar marks. Without anyone's knowledge, we have late-night chats, during which I listen for hours to his woeful stories. What are friends for? I cannot wait to see him. As a trailer pulls up beside my convalescence stall, my heart trembles with anticipation. "Roland, I'm here!" I call out, knowing that my knight tunes in and understands my every expression.

I ride home with a sense of well-being, free of my former discomfort. Once I realize that I have arrived at the Silver Saddle, I lift my head, look in the direction of the stalls, and neigh to my friends the news of my homecoming. Roland laughs, as he declares to the trailer driver: "He sounds like Ricky Ricardo, exclaiming 'Lucy, I'm home!'" Roland's quotation must be a human joke that I don't understand. I just give everyone a conciliatory nod.

To my disappointment, however, I discover that I must be on stall rest for a week. I live for Roland's daily visits, during which he feeds me hay, horse cookies, apples and carrots. While grooming me, my knight offers words of inspiration: "Rome wasn't built in a day, Areion. Brick by brick, we will build our dreams and dance one day in a beginners' dressage competition, acclaimed as winners! I am with you."[17]

One day, I hear Roland speaking with my first vet, Dr. Brant. Though I cannot understand the entire conversation, my ears perk up when I hear my name. Roland seems upset and, ever defending my cause, does not accept the doctor's "evasive" answers (once again, some words elude my understanding).

When my stitches are removed, I can, at last, graze for about a week. Then, Roland begins to walk me on a lead line. I still feel a little weak, but I am grateful for the joy of being home and walking without pain. Life's plan must be good for me now.

Soon, Roland receives clearance to ride with me, and I am filled with a sense of purpose and joy. I can almost smell the outdoors as it beckons to me. This is a perfect day to go riding, an ideal Sunday afternoon with my best friend. The sunshine and fresh air make me feel glad to be alive, and I am in good form, despite persistent pain in my foot. I choose to ignore all woes on this fine day. Nothing can keep me down. My discomfort seems to have eased a bit after surgery and I am less weighted down and able to roam. Roland senses that if he does not take me outside, I will get barn fever. He offers to take me grazing in the picnic campground area, a short distance from my stall. I can't wait, and my heart beats with excitement at the chance to graze in the sunlight.

As Roland leads me out of the barn, he takes care to pause for awhile, so that my eyes can adjust to the sun and the panoramic view. Humans and equines wind down after their weekend trail riding, clamoring to make their way around the farm. Like a welcoming nymph, the air touches my back and beckons me to celebrate my freedom. Heeding the call, I prepare to roll in the fragrant grass. I proceed to paw at the ground, loosen the soil, and step forward

---

[17]   Roland paraphrases John "Red" Pollard, portrayed by Tobey Maguire, in the movie *Seabiscuit* (2003).

to align all four of my legs together. I then raise my head, flex my forelegs, kneel on my pasterns and knees, tuck my hind legs under my body, and lower myself to the ground. "Life is good," I neigh loudly as I roll back and forth. Roland laughs as he watches me, fully understanding my natural inclinations, but warning me to be careful.

"Take it easy, Areion! When you get up, remember that you're on the lead line!" He calls.

Though I acknowledge Roland's warning, I choose not to rise immediately. I look up at the blue sky and admire the billowing clouds which, if I stare long enough, seem to form horse shapes. What an imagination I have! I wonder if humans play a similar game. Flies buzz all around me, as the grass sways in the breeze. I roll contentedly, as my heightened senses allow me to listen to nature's symphony. Then, I thrust my forelegs out in front of me, raise my forehand, and engage my hind legs so as to lift myself up. As I grunt, shake myself off, and kick out my hind legs, Roland steps to the side. I hear him tell me that he can't play with me like my equine buddies do, so I must temper my energy and enthusiasm. I neigh in reply, meaning that "I just can't help myself. I feel so good today." The following day proves to be just as fruitful and pain-free. When Roland comes by to see me, I lower my head and nudge him, indicating that I want to go for a ride. As usual, Roland takes my hint, and puts me on the nearby crossties at my friend Nacho's side. As Roland gathers his tack equipment, Nacho and I savor carrots and homemade horse cookie treats. Roland then brushes off my back and belly, cleans my hooves, and sprays an anti-bug mist over me. He then wraps my lower leg tendons for support, places a clean white pad on my back, pulls it up to my withers and, then, puts an English saddle on my back, securing it around my belly. He then unhooks me from the crossties and places the bridal over my head. The bridal has something on it which, Roland explains, is a so-called "nameplate."

Roland puts a bit in my mouth with a smear of peanut butter on it. Suddenly, I feel empowered. Finally, I have an identity! No one can mistake me for just "that horse" or "boy!" I have a name! I stand proudly with my head held high, not only to show the majesty of my stance but, also, to declare myself. Never again will I have to be someone's property, an owned commodity, beaten and kicked into submission. My heart and spirit belong only to me, and are beyond price. Humans may believe that we equines and other creatures of the earth are indifferent to cruelty, but nothing could be farther from the truth. We are living, breathing entities, whose main purpose is to please and to love.

As a feeling of strength pervades me, I am reminded of those fellow equines who, at this very moment, are being abused and neglected by unfit owners. In my past, I encountered many who were malnourished, not given proper water and sunlight; others writhed in pain from illnesses and injuries which went untreated; still others were sent to slaughter for no reason other than that they were no longer able to perform their tasks. I had been a cutting horse, and I know that when someone like I am becomes "useless" (as humans often say), life is over. I was just very fortunate that, thanks to my knight, I did not meet a similar fate.

Filled with gratitude, I am inspired to pay due tribute, in thought, to my fallen friends.

Take heart, good souls, the day is near
When humans will dispense with fear,
And love for just the sake of love,
Without the motives they think of,
Like money, fame, and fortune great.
The small things they'll appreciate.
For being heartfelt and true blue
Should not be just for very few.
Your lives have never been in vain,
Great spirits, rise above the pain!
Immortal you will always be.
May my example set you free!

My knight calls, and I return to the present moment. "Areion, listen to me, buddy! Are you ready to go for our ride?" As Roland and I leave the barn and enter the outdoor arena, my eyes adjust to the sun during my knight's intermittent pauses. He looks around for impending activity that can cause me to become frightened and rear up. Then, he stops at a small stoop, gets on my back, adjusts his boots in the stirrup, and grasps the reins.

"Remember, walk low and long, Areion," Roland gently instructs me.

My knight is strong and kind, and his respect for me makes me want to do my best and reward him with a pleasant ride. Many people at the barn stop to look in our direction. Someone calls out, "wow, you don't get to ride together very often, do you? Have fun! You look great!"

As I raise my head even higher, I catch a glimpse of Big Ben, the large draft horse who lives outside with the ponies, taking note. I feel like a performer.

"This is what it would be like to perform in a dressage competition, my friend!" Roland's voice resonates with pride and contentment.

Suddenly, Roland decides to trot, taps my sides with his boots, and begins to post, so as to spare my back and legs. He sits in the saddle only when my outside shoulder goes back. When we change reins, my knight maintains our unison by sitting down and rising in an uneven number of strides. Somehow, he always knows what is best for me—for both of us. The warm summer breeze allows my mane to flare out behind me. This must be what forever feels like. I wish that we could capture this moment, and never let it end.

Chapter 6

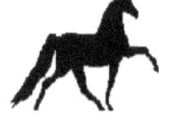

Joyful Engagements
(Roland's Narrative)

S itting in a cubicle, earning a living is not tantamount to enjoying every day moments, the act of actual living. In fact, the two engagements are entirely separate, especially when office pettiness and tedium factor into the mix. Each time I mention Areion to co-workers, very seldom do I receive a nod of understanding or empathetic friendship. No one truly fathoms how much he means to me and the nature of our deep connection.

I cannot begin—or even try—to explain how good it feels to ride with him out in the open air. No one would understand—and I cannot expect that of anyone caught up in mundane rituals. That is not to say that work is not important or that some people may actually enjoy rote tasks. Nothing is wrong with that, of course; but what is the purpose of poking fun at someone who wants to think outside of the box? If one has never experienced the closeness I have with Areion, descriptions fall on deaf ears. I cannot pretend that the nonchalance and ridicule with which I'm confronted at work does not hurt me; but, out in the sunshine with my equine confidante, it all doesn't matter. Areion seems to understand me. He has a comprehension that goes far beyond the spoken word. Who knows how much he and other horses really understand? Sometimes, when I look into his eyes, I see a timelessness, a profound knowledge that I don't discern often in human beings. I suspect that since he is close to the earth—a true product of it, he has secrets to which we bipeds are not privy.

I also feel, at times, that Areion peers into my soul. When I am lonely or afraid, I know that I can confide in him and receive his silent spirit wisdom, which speaks volumes. I know that he is so grateful and happy to have been rescued, and he shows me—literally with every step he takes.

Though I truly do not know what the future holds or whether we will be able to perform in a dressage competition, I constantly sense in my friend the willingness to try. He appreciates every move we make together—walks, trots and posts—which, to me, as well, are the most joyful engagements. Nothing compares to the time we spend together, which is like a healing salve for the continuous roughshod politicking of the office environment.

I wish that all horse owners who are privileged and fortunate enough to be in their presence would pay heed to the wisdom and beauty they confer. Every act of neglect and abuse directed toward them should toll the bell for humans, too; for we all breathe the same air and take the same course of life's progression and decline. Not one of us—neither animal nor human—is immune to life's alterations, and those who believe the contrary and live out their lives denigrating animals—some of the greatest of our world's resources—are in for rude awakenings. We are them and they are us. They cry and bleed as we do. They take joy in acts of kindness. I know, for Areion tells me. I think all of these thoughts during our couple of rides—and whenever we are joyfully engaged, just being together. I am so thankful for those times when Areion takes me out of myself and my sometimes narrow existence and shows me the splendor of greenery and sunshine. How I wish that all of such moments would endure!

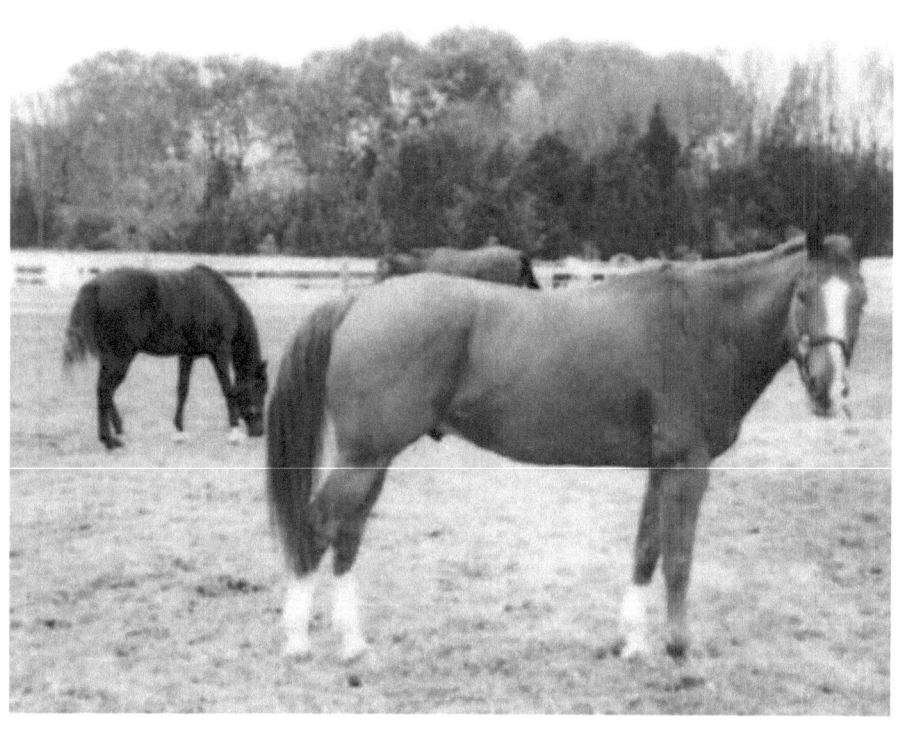

Chapter 7

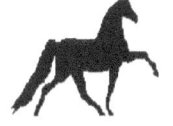

In and Out of Darkness
(Areion's Narrative)

*I*gnoring pain is never a wise decision for, sooner or later, one has to face the reality of what is, instead of what should be. I learn this lesson one day when Dr. Samuels' assistant comes to evaluate my condition, and trots me in a straight line. This is easy, I sigh to myself. However, I hear and observe Roland speaking, with knitted brow, to the assistant.

"Aren't you going to run him in a circle?"

"No, he is fine," the assistant states coldly.

"Is that the full extent of the exam?" my knight inquires eagerly.

"Yes, he is fine," the assistant replies and exits quickly.

As Roland attempts to ride me again, I feel a familiar pain. Something is not right, I say to myself. Roland notices that I am still coming up short and have a hard time with left turns. What can, possibly, be the matter now? Where is our miracle? I ask Roland in my spirit. My knight's thoughts are far away, as he tries to shape our destiny. Suddenly, he dismounts and speaks with his sister through a strange device which practically all humans own. I feel anxious as I witness my knight's eyes well with water. He does his best to conceal emotion.

"Connie, I am at my wit's end. My only hope is Dr. Patty Hogan, whom I saw on television yesterday. She is the gifted vet who saved Smarty Jones from a nearly devastating skull fracture and eye injuries. Maybe, she can help my Areion."

I begin to tremble, sensing that I must endure yet another vet visit. Roland explains that we will see a famous doctor in Clarksburg, New Jersey. Maybe, this is my chance, I think to myself, investing faith in my knight. Time seems to be endless, as I await the moment of departure. In the meantime, Roland transfers me to a more spacious end of the barn. All of my new barn mates provide encouragement, especially Bello, the Andalusian stallion of the flowing black mane, Tristan, the lone, big warmblood (who, except for Roland's carrots, does not receive the grace of human kindness), and Schatz, the beautiful black- and-white art-deco stallion, whose kind nature always makes me smile. Dominique's Nacho, who misses my company, sends over a friendly neigh-borly greeting.

Within two days, a trailer arrives and my knight tries to comfort me as he puts on my shipping boots. "I am here, Areion, and you will be treated properly now." In reply, I raise my long neck, feigning confidence, as I do not wish to compound my knight's fears with my own. Soon, we arrive at a place called the "New Jersey Equine Clinic," which displays a sign outside: "Congratulations, Smarty Jones!" A kind, attractive lady emerges from the facility to welcome me, with rain pouring down around us. Introducing herself as "Dr. Patty," she pets my head and neck, making me feel safe and confident. In the doctor's presence, I am impervious to the storm, a metaphor for my inner torrent.

Dr. Patty trots me and performs a nerve block, to which I am very accustomed. Dr. Patty and my knight speak for about an hour, in which Roland learns of her history with and love for horses. Clearly, she has a fervent desire to serve us. Her expertise, perceptiveness and commitment have no parallel.

"Don't ever abandon him," the doctor gently admonishes my knight. "He has nice movements for an appendix, and would make a good beginner's dressage horse. I am going to take x-rays and keep him overnight." Roland leaves, reassuring me of his abiding support. The next day, as I rest from my exam in a holding room, I overhear Dr. Patty speaking to my best friend, whose voice I always recognize.

"The x-rays show that Areion has navicular degeneration in both feet, more acutely on the left side, which accounts for his limp and pain. There is, as well, an old fracture in Areion's right knee that has gone untreated in the past. We are very fortunate that the bone fragments have not moved and, given the lapse of time between the fracture incident and the present, most likely will not cause damage." Dr. Patty's voice is measured, inflected with compassion.

My knight manages to ask: "What can we do now?"

"I will leave the knee fracture alone, and perform surgery on both feet," Dr. Patty says decisively.

Roland concedes, trusting in Dr. Patty's care of me. "She is an artist-practitioner, a graduate of the University of Pennsylvania at New Bolton. You could not be in better hands, Areion," my knight declares. I remain at the clinic for five days, in which I receive care never before experienced. My comfortable stall and daily diet of hay and treats provide enormous contentment and security. My only lack: the soothing presence of my greatest human companion. When Roland comes to take me home, I walk proudly out of the trailer, in spite of a limp on my left side. By my demeanor, I declare myself to be a steed worthy of recognition. The barn's surroundings seem to echo my inner conviction.

As I walk through the center of the facility, I witness a splendid sight. The barn's barren, arid atmosphere has transformed into a tropical paradise. In my absence, my knight planted flowers and exotic plants everywhere, constructed a patio for the trail riders, cut the grass and provided drainage for the horses. I cannot not believe that the mud is gone! The poles are freshly painted, and there is a new sitting area outside of the barn. I am proud of Roland's ingenuity.

Everyone in and around the Silver Saddle admires my knight's devotion, dubbing him "Mr. Silver Saddle." Even Dr. Brant has a kind word for him. On one particular morning, as Roland grooms me, the vet approaches and observes:

"No one would care for this horse as you do." Dr. Brant walks quickly past.

My knight turns to me and pets my head.

"It may take awhile for people to acknowledge us, Areion, but when our time comes, look out world!"

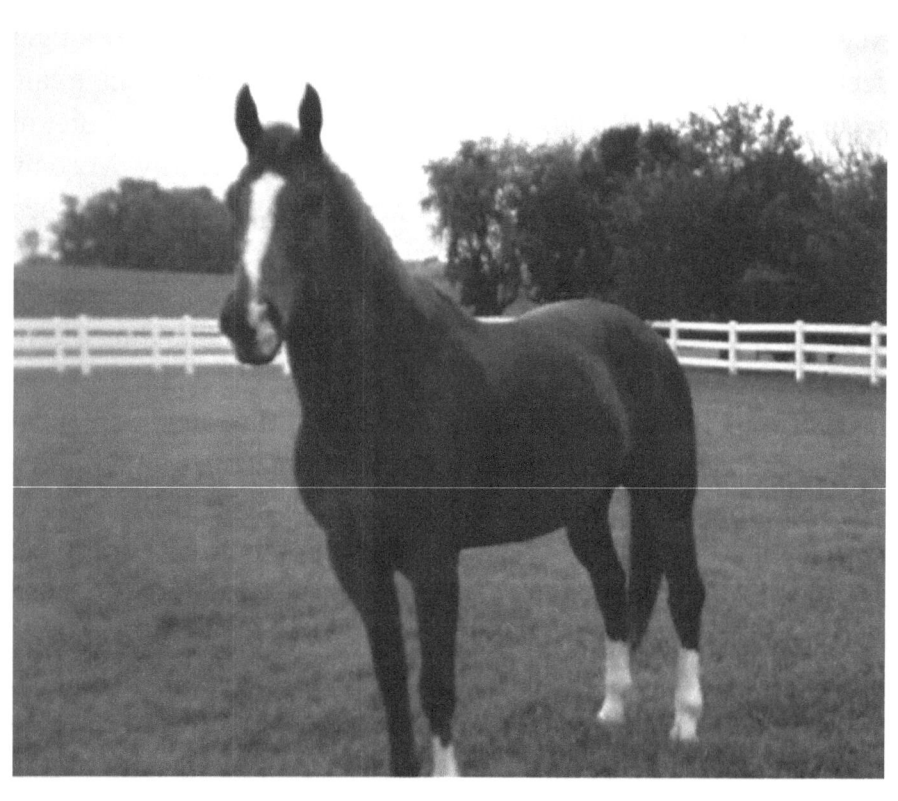

Chapter 8

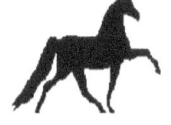

Destiny's Two Faces
(Roland's Narrative)

*L*ife's bittersweet roller coaster ride only serves to embolden me and my intrepid companion, who has become my rock. The more hurdles we encounter, the higher we learn to jump.

After the second surgery, Areion goes on stall rest again for about a week. Dr. Patty believes in brief convalescence time, and we agree with her judgment. A horse needs to run, breathe in fresh air and frolic in green pastures. When Dr. Patty renders clearance for hand walking, she reaffirms her assessment of Areion's good mind and spirit, and his potential for beginner's dressage training. Our hearts resonate with the prospect of a new chapter. Ever placid and accepting of life's vicissitudes, Areion's only wish is to be loved and to love.

Fate steps in once more, however. While at the gym, I suffer a herniated disc, necessitating surgery and a four- to six-month recovery period. Out of work and unable to drive, I visit Areion as much as possible, while deferring to my trusted friends, Dominique and Gerry, to keep an eye on him.

My state of incapacity once again finds a parallel in the life of my star-crossed companion. When I arrive for a visit one day, I observe him limping. How can this be? I think to myself, wondering what may have occurred. Under strict supervision, Areion can walk outside for only a few minutes at a time. Is it possible that someone allowed him to run out on his own? Did I not leave specific instructions for his care? My mind races, as Areion looks at me, as if to declare, "I know, destiny has two faces. One day, she smiles, and the next, she frowns." He nuzzles me, endeavoring to offer comfort.

"If it were not for you, my friend, I hardly could look destiny squarely in the eyes," I whisper softly.

After two days, with the kind assistance of my trainer, Jane, we return to Dr. Patty, who diagnoses Areion with a deep-flexor-tendon tear,[18] which bears out my suspicion of negligence.

"I am not giving up on a creature whose only wish is to live and to love me," I reply, choking back a wellspring of feeling. I believe in a comeback—for both of us."

"So do I," says Dr. Patty, soothingly. "A six- to nine-month recovery is required for this type of injury. Areion cannot run out or engage in any protracted activity,"

Upon leaving the office, I plan to retain a local vet, Dr. Katherine Alsace, who performs a series of ultrasound exams to determine the size of the tear (revealed to be about that of a quarter).

With such a malaise, Areion has to be hand walked during the day to avert stir-craziness until I arrive in the evening. In what I term "the cartoon incident," one of the hand walkers, professing to be experienced, receives the shock of her life. Areion spots a deer, rears up, and drags her along as he runs back to his stall. Somehow, the bewildered girl does not let go and looks like an animated doll, as she trails behind him. Fortunately, the incident leaves her unscathed, as I begin the rehiring process. Susan Villani from Readington, New Jersey, an experienced barn owner, proves to be a perfect companion, who comes three to four days per week.

Areion's daily regime of vitamins and supplements (eighteen pills per day, in total) makes feeding a chore. At times, my clever friend tries to separate his food from the pills, but I manage to keep this habit in check. I also maintain a routine of soaking Areion's foot and treating the tendon with infrared laser therapy. As a result of meticulous care, the tear shows signs of healing

---

[18] The deep flexor tendon runs over the back of the knee in the carpal canal and is held in position by the carpal check ligament.

in the seventh months subsequent to surgery, much sooner than expected.

As we both convalesce, I observe a new trainer at the barn, Kati Regan, an employee of a renowned international dressage trainer. She has been hired to instruct Bello, the Andalusian stallion, in dressage. Observing her casually, I am too timid to approach her. When I finally summon the courage to address Kati about training, I receive an amicable reply:

"Sure! We will work out a payment schedule and, when Areion gets clearance from the vet, we will begin."

"Thank you! We can't wait!" I extend my hand, incredulous at her down-to-earth nature.

Soon, I receive clearance from Dr. Alsace for Areion to commence dressage training.[19] Kati puts him under saddle, building muscle strength with walks around the arena, using special tack equipment to keep his head "low and long." Later, with uncommon grace, my determined friend goes diagonally across the arena, appearing to float on air. By his gaze, I can tell that he is living a dream.

I also begin lessons with designated school horses whom Kati had trained for such purposes. I use a lunge line, which Kati holds as I travel in a circle, posting up and down to the horse's rhythm.

---

[19] Dressage is likened to ballet and gymnastics on horseback, involving the aesthetically beautiful, harmonious movements of horse and rider, which demonstrate flexibility, poise and strength. The first practitioners of this method of "dance" were the ancient Greeks, who believed in preparing their horses for battle according to strict universal laws and principles. Their aim was to have the horse submit to the rider's will, without disruption of natural grace and flow. The Greek commander, Xenophon (ca. 431-355 B.C.), wrote the first recorded work on classical dressage, entitled Hippike(The Art of Horsemanship). The tradition then spread to Rome, Spain and, later, Austria and Germany. One of the most advanced movements in dressage is piaffe, a highly controlled, cadenced trot.

Then, I execute balance drills, with both arms straight out in front of me, posting in a trot, without grasping the reigns.

"Feet beneath you!" Kati instructs, emphasizing the importance of a perpendicular seating position. "In the unlikely event that the horse goes out from under you, you will land straight on your feet," she explains. Team Areion's timing is good and, as in all instances, synchronized. We just about progress to the point of riding together, when crushing news reaches us regarding Kati's forced departure. Apparently, her work with Bello brings him to a dressage show but, when Kati discovers that she cannot take the trip, Betty summarily fires her.

"If she goes, I go!" I address Betty with deep unrest. "The quality of care here has declined immeasurably. Yesterday, I found stickers in Areion's hay, and the feed quality is not up to par." Indignation rises within me.

"If you don't approve of conditions here, you can leave," Dave states unapologetically, as he walks up beside me.

"You must give thirty days' notice."

In the interim, I unsuccessfully travel from barn to barn, each time beset with rejection, either due to lack of room or facilities to care for Areion. As I ruminate on the two faces of destiny and my next course of action, I am reminded of the quote "[f]or everything you have missed, you have gained something else and, for everything you gain, you lose something else."[20] I employ ingenuity to help fate along and, in little time, Areion finds a home at a quaint barn in Kingwood.

---

[20]   Ralph Waldo Emerson (1803-1882), American essayist and poet.

Chapter 9

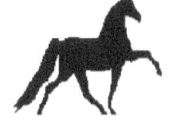

Treading On Uncertain Ground
(Areion's Narrative)

ince my younger days, I have had several trust issues with human beings, owing to many hardships and strains placed upon me. Fears still envelope me as a result and, from time to time, residual memories surface. The stories are too long and painful for me to revisit but, now, thanks to Roland, I can leave the past behind and hold my head to the sun.

On this particular day, however, unpleasant recollections revive, as a two- horse trailer comes to take me away from the Silver Saddle. I attempt to ask where I am going, but no one understands me. As ever, I decide to invest faith in my devoted knight who, after allowing me to say goodbye to friends, ushers me into a trailer, assuring me that he is at my side. That is all I need to know, and nothing else matters. When I hear Nacho protest, I answer, in my spirit, that all will be well.

"This is far too small," I hear Roland commenting on the two-horse trailer. "I specifically requested a larger trailer for Areion, due to his fears of backing down ramps or over objects."

"The barn owner did not feel it was necessary," replies Tamara, the driver, also a staff trainer at the barn.

We proceed to ride in a space of about eight feet, barely room for me to breathe. How can anyone expect my sixteen-hand, two-inch, twelve-hundred-pound frame to fit into, not to mention exit from, the trailer? I ask myself.

Upon my arrival home, I feel tension rising within me. Realizing that I must back up off of the trailer ramp, I categorically refuse. My anxieties concerning backward motions down ramps and over other similar obstructions cannot be expressed in human terms. My gentle knight's coaxing with carrots, cookies, and apples do not serve to calm me, as I remain with all four hooves firmly planted on the ground. After a full hour, I finally decide to turn around and, with the force of my weight behind me, bend the divider and throw my knight from the trailer ramp. I topple out with him, fortunately uninjured. As I collect myself and gaze about, I look for Roland, who stands beside me, laughing. "I feel as if I have been squeezed from a toothpaste tube!" he exclaims. Without understanding Roland's meaning, I am, simply, glad that both of us are in one piece. Roland introduces me to a new barn and walks me around. I am impressed by the barn's external appearance and even more delighted when I enter to see my new, windowed stall. "This is a nice place!" I neigh blissfully, as I roll on my back. My knight senses that I am happy, and his heart lifts, as well. Somehow, we always manage to be in unison.

On my second day at the new barn, pangs of nostalgia for my former barn dissipate, as I bid Nacho well in my heart, never to forget him or any of my other equine companions. I make new friendships, particularly with Flannery, a beautiful ivory horse, with whom I truly run free. We neigh together (just as some humans sing duets), prance about, and get into mischief. One day, when we play roughly and knock over a nylon separating fence, Roland comes and gently admonishes me, with a twinkle in his eye.

"You are like an errant schoolboy, Areion!" I realize that I must keep away from fences, resisting the contrary temptation when I am with Flannery. All in all, I am content, and my feet seem to be healing well.

Then, situations begin to decline when I train with the barn's staff trainer, Tamara, an eventer, who handles me quite differently from Kati at the Silver Saddle. Roland paid her to take me out a given number of times, but she failed to do so. Oh, how I miss my Kati saying: "Hello, Mr. Areion!" She certainly knows how to make me feel special. Every night, I signal to her, in the spirit, to visit me. Employing her own techniques, Tamara manages to reverse everything I accomplished with Kati. Soon, my muscle tone breaks down from improper riding. Though my head should be long and curved, Tamara holds my reigns in such a way that my head assumes a shortened, forward extension, and my motions become choppy, less fluid. Soon, I feel that my coffin bone[21] begins to deteriorate, and I come up short again on the left side. As my condition progressively worsens, my knight's concerns escalate. I observe his unrest and try to comfort him. He teaches me something called "hugging," which involves lowering and placing my head on his shoulder at the command "give me a hug." This motion seems to soothe our anxieties and affirm our unflagging commitment to one another, to my healing and, ultimately, our dream of dancing in a beginner's dressage show. I shudder to think where I would be without my steadfast knight and our shared goals!

As any human, equine, or other creature may well imagine, I loathe taking supplements and all manner of medical intervention. Reluctantly, I must submit to everything from B12 injections, chiropractic adjustments, and acupuncture, to all of which Roland subjects me purely out of love. Without signs of improvement, x-rays become necessary, and Dr. Alsace, to whose face I have grown accustomed, comes to take them.

My sorrow is mitigated one afternoon by a surprise visit from Kati and Dominique, my best human friends from the Silver Saddle. The words, "Hello, Mr. Areion!" reach my hearing and almost effectuate a cure, while Dominique's caress makes my heart light. I overhear Kati telling Roland that she plans to move to Florida, where she will work as a barn manager for a former U.S. Olympic Gold Medalist in dressage.

"Barbara is such a lovely woman," Kati explains, "and I am looking forward to my new job."

"Congratulations! I cannot pretend that Areion and I will not be sorry to lose you, Kati," my knight replies, with more than a little melancholy in his voice. "You have been an invaluable friend and instructor."

---

[21] The coffin bone is encased inside of the horse's hoof.

"Don't worry, Roland. We will stay in touch," Kati answers reassuringly. "Please keep me posted on Areion's progress."

"Roland!" Just as she is about to leave, Dominique runs up to my knight.

"Nacho has been moved to a nice backyard barn, and he likes his new home very much! I go there every day to take care of him." Dominique's eyes glisten with contentment.

"I will tell Areion." Roland smiles widely. He does not have to tell me, for my heart already beats joyfully at the news.

When my Kati and Dominique depart, and I am left to divert my attention, I visit the other horses in the barn. My helpful neigh-bors empathize with my plight and ease my burden. As we graze together, I overhear a disturbing conversation, the substance of which pertains to me. Yet again, my knight goes on the defensive.

"You have to buy a round pen and a run-in shelter, so that Areion can remain outside," Jackie, the barn owner, declares.

"Not for any purpose in the world will I keep Areion outside," my knight insists. "While in my care, he has never lived outside, and he will not begin now."

"You should retire him, you know or, otherwise, put him down," Jackie states matter-of-factly. "Horses like that just . . . ."

My knight does not allow her to continue. "This conversation is making me ill. I have to go." Roland departs, with his head lowered, appearing to hold his stomach. From my vantage point, I see his determined glance. Clearly, he has a plan, but I do not know his thoughts. His spirit is closed to all communication.

The next day, two strangers come to remove me from my stall. Frantically, I look about for my knight, who is nowhere to be found. I tremble inside but, somehow, the gracious pair seems intent on my well-being. Has Roland abandoned me? I reflect for a moment and, then, submit to the humans' gentle commands.

"Come on Areion," the petite, soft-spoken lady says. She is, obviously, very accustomed to horses. "I'm Liz, and this is Mike. We are going to make you strong and well again." She points to a tall, imposing gentleman with a deeply compassionate, competent expression. I imagine that he can do anything! I affirm to myself. I am in good hands, but where, oh where, is my knight?

When Roland comes the next day, I decide to be silent, keeping my head down. My knight tempts me with treats, and I return to myself again, realizing that he always intends the best for me. I should have known that he would return.

Slowly, Mike trains me on a device known as a "water treadmill," designed to tone and strengthen my muscles. Mike habituates me to the treadmill by walking down a long aisle up to the device and, then, onto it, by degrees. Mike controls the speed of the treadmill and the water within. Each time I respond to his commands to walk, Mike rewards me with carrots. I can do this! I try to convince myself. At first, the water rises about two to three inches and, then, gradually, with each session, rises up to my chest. The low-impact exercise for my tendons and joints allows me to move freely, unrestrained, and I bask in the illusion that I no longer tread on uncertain ground.

Chapter 10

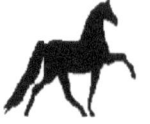

Living In The Moment
(Roland's Narrative)

One afternoon, I decide to take a day off from work to meet Dr. Alsace at High Brass Farm, Areion's new home. Filled with anticipation, I wonder what his recent x-rays will reveal. We have been through so much together, and we require some positive news. When we all assemble, Mike trots Areion down the aisle of the rehab center, so that Dr. Alsace can evaluate his progress after his two-week water treadmill therapy. My heart pulsates rapidly with the hope that lameness does not surface again. Ever valiant, Areion does not disappoint, trotting gracefully down the aisle without visible signs of pain. His movements belie the cold underlying truth about to be unveiled.

As we advance into the all-purpose room (i.e. a combination kitchen, supply room, and visiting veterinarian's workspace), Dr. Alsace beckons me to a lighted wallcase to view the x-rays. The presence of Liz and Mike helps to mitigate my increasing anxiety. My heart sinks, as Dr. Alsace points out that Areion's left foot has deteriorated markedly, his coffin bone in decline, trying to adhere to his navicular bone.

"We have never seen anything like this," Liz and Mike comment, almost in unison.

I summon strength to speak for my hero and myself, so long in the clutches of fate's unrelenting hand.

"Is there anything we can do to stop the process of degeneration?" I ask haltingly. "Areion has the heart and spirit of a champion, even though conventional 'wisdom' devalues his life by comparing him, strictly in monetary terms, to five-hundred-thousand-dollar Grand Prix dressage horses. My Areion has such a desire to make the best of adversity, to overcome the odds, and I am not prepared to break his spirit or restrain a life which longs to reach its greatest potential. Our road has been long but, in my heart, I feel that we have not gone the full distance."

Vanquishing all the shadows of our past, I finish my plea with more conviction than I have ever entertained. Dr. Alsace concedes and focuses her attention on treatment.

"Areion must create his own synovial fluids, so as to lubricate the coffin and navicular bone areas," she explains. "I will prescribe Pentoxifylline to increase circulation. Areion must take eighteen tablets per day. He also must undergo a series of Adequan injections to aid in the production of new cartilage and promote repair."

"We can begin immediately, Doctor," I state decisively. "There is no time like the present."

Doctor Alsace proceeds to sedate Areion by injecting his coffin bone. As Areion lapses in and out of consciousness, I hold his head, all the while speaking to him.

"Fight your fight, Areion! You cannot lose. We are together," I command my hero, stroking him.

To signify understanding, Areion opens his eyes ever so slightly, while my own fill with tears. I assure him of his impending well-being, through me.

"I will be your eyes, ears, and voice, my friend. No obstacle is too insurmountable where loves dwells and all things become possible," I whisper. Thus, we go along until, a few weeks after his treatment with Dr. Alsace, Areion contracts a bad cold and must be quarantined at the main barn annex. Despite the sweltering summer heat, Areion cannot bathe. During this period, his loneliness is profound and, so, I take daily half-days from work to visit and tend to him, wiping his nose and placing cold towels on his face. My hero watches me silently, in gratitude, with unflinching devotion. As we await negative laboratory test results, the slow progression of days seems endless. Areion only can walk out to graze, and we just revel in each other's company.

On one summer evening, I observe Areion in much better form, and I decide to lead him out to a big, open field. Standing with his characteristic pride and tall stature, my friend gazes out, wishing to be a horse, free to run with the wind. His spirit calls out:

"Let me go, Roland, just let me go!"

I glance quickly around the farm and, thankfully, find no one in sight.

"For all that you have been through, you deserve this my friend," I murmur, in hushed tones, as if someone were eavesdropping.

Always have I nurtured Areion not only to be my partner in learning dressage but, also, as a creature of the Earth, of unrestrained motion and power. Turnout is important for training and performance horses alike, so that their minds and bodies can be supple and more resistant to injuries. Sadly, some "high-end" horses never experience turnout due to their owner's fear of injury. Therefore, they cannot develop necessary bone mass and agility. I witnessed such practices first-hand after visiting many barns, taking classes and reading texts. Not to allow Areion the joy of his natural inclinations would be cruel, I think to myself.

"Dr. Alsace, Liz and Mike would not approve of what I am about to do." I lower my head to speak in Areion's ear. "But if you don't tell, I won't."

As I remove Areion's lead line, he trots down the hill and runs like the wind, kicking up his back legs, throwing his head about and neighing more loudly than a herd of elephants. At last, all of his suppressed energy bursts forth. As the wind begins to pick up with an impending rainstorm, my hero runs in the tall grass, stretching every muscle and sinew, like a child exiting school for summer vacation. The cool rain descends, as Areion takes his fill of grass, never wanting the moment to end.

"Areion, come back in!" I call, not wishing to overstep boundaries for too long. My hero is impervious to such restrictions, however. Freedom is far too sweet. Suddenly, Mike comes toward me, speaking reproachfully:

"You should not allow Areion to roam like that."

"I know, Mike, but he just wants to be as God made him, free to run, to graze and feel the wind," I explain, holding fast to every justification.

"He will be very sore tomorrow," Mike cautions.

"We have to take chances, Mike. Areion's freedom is worth the price," I reply.

Such is the joy of living in the moment, tapping the full extent of capacity, unshackled by opinion or judgment. Such is the bliss of being who we are, exquisitely uncompromising and free!

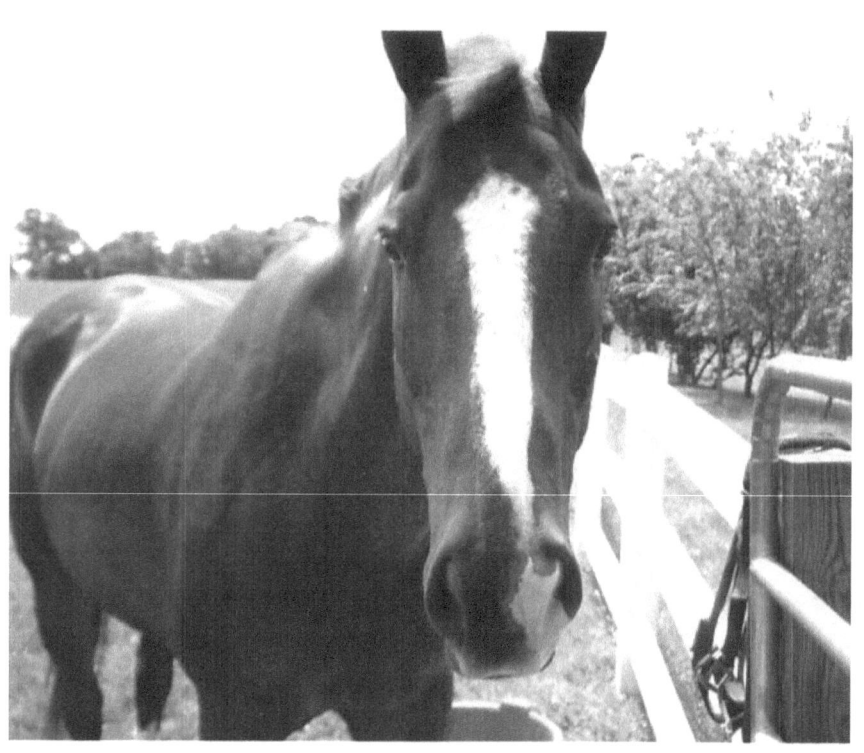

Chapter 11

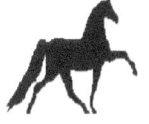

My Four-Leaved Clover
(Areion's Narrative)

My knight truly knows how to make my life worthwhile. He took a great risk in turning me out; but freedom (which has no price) is well worth a few days of convalescence. I go stir-crazy when I have to look at the four walls of my stall all the time. I would rather go searching for clovers, my favorite leaves.

Luckily, my cold has gone, and the doctor told Roland that I am free to reunite with my friends at the rehab center and begin water treadmill therapy again. I have missed Mike and Liz very much. I should mention that Liz is a renowned rider and has innumerable ribbons (I have not seen them first-hand, of course, but my knight has told me about them). How fortunate I am to be in such care!

I need a good farrier, and Mike refers Roland to Scott Previte, a skillful, knowledgeable man, who loves horses. After examining my foot, he tells my knight that I have a mild case of White Line Disease[22] which, if left untreated, can cause complications (such as the breakdown of the hoof's weight-support system, a foot infection or, in severe cases, lameness). Sometimes, I hear Scott consulting with my vet through the strange device which practically every human owns. I am very popular, I think to myself.

Soon, Scott constructs proper shoes for me and, with my monthly injections, my foot continues to feel nimble and pain-free. I revel in times when my knight spends long days at the center, confiding in me, reflecting on life, as we trot in the fresh air. I graze in the sun,

---

[22]   White Line Disease is a condition involving deterioration of a horse's hoof, causing it to have a dry, brittle appearance.

as Roland watches takeoffs of huge sky-vehicles from the airport next door. So vast and formidable, the world sometimes overwhelms me, as so many things elude my understanding. In particular, I fail to comprehend humans' inhumanity to themselves and to other creatures. My knight tells me of his tribulations in the workplace, where people do not empathize with his attachment to me. They make fun of our closeness and the fact that I have endured so many hardships.

"We have to hope for a miracle," Roland says, looking at me lovingly. "Sometimes, I believe that all of our difficulties have been a bad dream, from which we someday will awaken; but we cannot give up."

"Please do not worry, my Brother." I speak in my spirit, soothingly, as I trot to a field of clover.

"Areion, there are many clovers in this field but, somewhere, if we look deeply and long enough, we will find the four-leaved charm, which brings good luck," my knight explains.

I continue to graze in the clover, as Roland's thoughts trail off. Suddenly, he looks down and exclaims, with joy:

"Do you see, Areion? You have found the prize, the four-leaved clover! Do you understand? We must keep hope alive, and we can find the treasure if we only look—inside of ourselves."

Roland smiles at my neighing and grunting, realizing that the magic of the four-leaved clover rings true for both of us, a metaphor for himself, a graceful summation of our life together.

Chapter 12

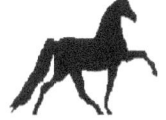

Life's Tests
(Roland's Narrative)

*T*he soundness of Areion's gait sets me to thinking about his future and our training in beginner's freestyle dressage. Timing is of the essence, and I take a day from work to meet Dr. Alsace at High Brass Farm. When the doctor arrives, I attempt to contain my heightened sense of Areion's well-being and the ability to realize our dream. Areion's spirit radiates and affirms, "I am ready to begin!"

As I trot Areion outside in circles, Dr. Alsace and Mike observe that he still comes up slightly short on the left side.

"Let's go to the indoor arena and test him on the soft sand and dust footing," Mike suggests.

As we proceed to our destination from the rehab center to the upper barn, we pass fields and pastures, where other horses graze. With his customary dignity, Areion lifts his head and neighs to his friends, as if to say, "I'm testing today. Wish me luck!"

The soft surface of the indoor arena proves to be forgiving to Areion's feet and, at Dr. Alsace's request, we trot in a big circle and, then, in different directions, at a brisk pace. Finally, we circle once more, stopping in front of Mike and Dr. Alsace, both of whom beam at Areion's progress.

"There is no sign of lameness, on the forgiving surface of this arena," Dr. Alsace comments. Mike shakes his head, with pride and incredulity.

"Never would any stranger, not knowing what Areion has endured, believe that he has had so many problems."

"We did it, Areion!" I shout, as I pat my hero on the neck. "Good Boy! YES!" My mind begins to wander, as I plan our next step toward fulfillment of our mutual goal. Beginner's freestyle dressage lies in our reach, I tell myself.

Life's tests intervene, however (of a different nature in the human realm), when a dispute arises at work, instigated by my company's assistant vice president. One afternoon, he decides to end my twenty-year term of devoted service. Sitting in the cubicle directly behind me, he monitors one of my calls to and from the vet regarding Areion, and reports back to my Director. She, in turn, questions my actions, which I vehemently defend: "Areion is my family, valued just as much as any human being. If your grandchildren call, will you be as intolerant of yourself as you are of me?" Impervious to reason, the director defers to the assistant vice president, who relays the entire scenario to people in the home office. What sort of human being would do this?

One month after the incident, my director calls me in to meet with her and the human resources representative from Chicago, both of whom advise me that I am part of a workforce reduction and will remain with the company until early December. All at once, the full impact of injustice reaches me. My heart drops, as I realize that no longer will I be able to meet the costs of Areion's board and treatment at High Brass Farm, where he has made such marked progress.

As to the loss of my job, I reach the conclusion that the decision to terminate me has been based on personal choice, rather than reasoned necessity. Containing my emotion and desire to react, I take solace in knowing that, at least, I have my Areion.

With diminished financial resources, I decide to move Areion quickly from High Brass to another barn. Time and again in my search for a place to stay, I encounter discrimination against my friend, due to his past physical condition. Lack of compassion surfaces most glaringly at one barn, where the owner tells me that he will request our departure after one month's down time or lack of performance and will impose a penalty for each week of poor health. Such are the cruelties of human business practices in an industry which often flagrantly disregards heartbeats behind dollar signs.

After many disappointments, a quaint barn, closer to home in Branchburg, New Jersey, comes to my attention. The owner, Darlene, appears to be compassionate, receptive to our presence, and compliant with my request to supplement the outdoor arena with sand and stone dust, at my own expense. I emphasize that the place must conduce to Areion's walking, riding, and training, best accomplished on soft surfaces. With reasonable board and large stalls, our future here seems promising.

Mike awaits me with Areion for his pickup at High Brass Farm, where I arrive with Darlene and her friend, Judith, who generously offers her trailer. With the drop-off of another horse on the way, our trip seems endless. We finally arrive in the vicinity as nightfall's curtain begins to descend. Just then, the truck's rear brake malfunctions.

"Life is a test. It is only a test. If this had been our actual life, we would have been given better instructions," I quip, attempting levity. With temperatures dropping and our protracted time on the road, I decide to call Mike, who can fix anything. His masterful mechanic skills will pull us through, I assure myself, doubtful that I am not thinking aloud. Within minutes, Mike appears.

"The brake cylinder is bad. Braking fluid is leaking." Mike gives a definitive diagnosis. "I have a funny feeling in the pit of my stomach that this move is not right for Areion. Too many obstacles are blocking our intended path. The break is a metaphor for impending hardships to come." I speak in Judith's direction, as though I were a fortune teller.

"Wait! don't worry! My boyfriend has a truck. I will ask him to come and haul the trailer." Judith approaches me, as she takes out her cell phone.

After about an hour's wait, during which we painstakingly hook the trailer to the truck, we discover that there are only three seats for four people.

"I will ride in the trailer's dressing room," I offer.

"Absolutely not!" Darlene and Judith speak at once.

The ill feeling in my stomach continues to rise, as I fight my instincts to take Areion back to High Brass Farm. If I had the money, I would listen to my inner voice, but that call must take a back seat to pragmatism. I contemplate quietly, then raise my head to see Areion resisting his climb into the trailer. Perhaps, destiny is trying to tell him something, as well.

"Come on, boy!" Mike takes hold of my friend, as if by way of bidding farewell and wishing him good luck. "You're a good egg, Areion!" Mike calls out after boarding him.

I manage to board, restraining my tears, as I recall our enjoyable time at High Brass and the friendships we established there. "We will miss you," I whisper, almost inaudibly. Areion nods. Somehow he always hears me. As we head to Darlene's barn, night enshrouds us like a tarp, temporarily shielding us from an uncertain future.

Chapter 13

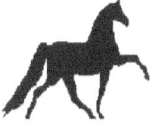

To Sleep, Perchance To Dream[23]
(Areion's Narrative)

My knight has been very troubled and senses my reluctance about going to another barn. In truth, I feel that the lady has misrepresented her barn knowledge and level of care for creatures like me. What can we do now? Roland wants the best for me, and we share a mutual dream for my ultimate well-being and our debut dressage performance. Oh, world, what do you have in store for us? Am I to be treated like property, chattel to be mishandled at someone's whim? In spite of myself, I am downcast. Never have I felt so physically sound, yet so unsure of my fate, tentative in the promise of a joyful future.

I observe Roland watching me in the trailer's video camera. He customarily checks on me, and I do not wish to worry him. In fact, I am, truly, well. I stand up straight, without any sign of discomfort, all the way to my new home. Inside, however, I feel the onset of an inexplicable, profound melancholy, which no one ever will detect. I hide my feelings well. When we arrive, I turn around and exit the trailer, taking care not to squeeze my knight out of it like "toothpaste" (whatever that is!).

For the first time in a long while, I am afraid of the darkness. I think of my former stall in Oklahoma, very long ago, where I lived as a cutting horse, considered 'a no one,' when my mind served as my sole refuge. Now, I am really alive, but upon whose time clock? Roland looks tired, as he begins to unload some tack boxes and feed.

"I will return tomorrow in the early afternoon to bring more of Areion's gear," he says, as he pats my neck.

---

23   A quote from Shakespeare's *Hamlet* in a famous soliloquy (III, i, 65-68).

"There is so much that I wish to tell you, my knight," I neigh, as he walks out. "Our time may never come!" I manage to conceal despair, evident only to the starry sky.

The next day, Roland arrives, preoccupied with unloading tack boxes, which can hardly fit into the small available spaces. I surmise that this is not a working barn and the lady, Darlene (whose name I eventually overhear), has limited nurturing skills, which I glean from her approach with me. As she shows my knight around the barn, I hear him speak to me in the spirit.

"We should not have come, my friend. We have to get out of here quickly."

My mind races back to our time at High Brass Farm, when Roland turned me out and I ran with the wind. How I wish to do that again! I feel that I will be here forever, cooped up and, possibly, treated poorly. My symptoms will resurface if we do not act immediately. No doubt, Roland reads my mind and, as usual, comes to my rescue. My ears perk up to hear my knight's words, as he stands beside me and secretly uses the strange device which practically every human owns.

"Kevin, I must speak with you. My original plan to board Areion with you after High Brass should have taken place, after all. I appreciate your knowledge of horses, and I love the beautiful barn constructed from trees on your property. I hesitated, at first, simply because of the long commute. Now, however, my mind is made up. I do not have a good feeling about where we are now, and we have to leave as soon as possible. The only problem is that I cannot get a trailer until the end of this week, and today is only Wednesday."

For a horse, time is eternal. "The end of this week" may signal the beginning of any moment, and each moment contains lifetimes. My Kati gives me countless years each time she says: "Hello, Mr. Areion!" Dominique bestows forever when she pats my head, and my knight confers everything is his very being. Sometimes, however, one moment can point toward time's end.

After the new dawn, my knight returns to find me in a hard, unforgiving paddock, filled with more dirt than those on the other side of the barn, where Darlene's own horses live in the soft grass. Despite my cataracts, I spot my knight's pale, dismayed visage.

"Why is Areion there?" Without awaiting Darlene's answer, Roland decidedly takes his tack equipment from the barn, loads it onto his truck, and leaves. Little does he know what occurred in his absence, how much my foot smarts, more than ever before. I can barely walk.

Upon my knight's return, I hear Darlene ask: "What is wrong with your horse?"

"Why? I told you of his past condition. What has happened?" Roland asks excitedly.

"He was limping very badly when he came in." Darlene replies, almost nonchalantly.

Upon approaching my stall, Roland breathes heavily and looks as though he is about to collapse. Recognizing my advanced debilitation, he slowly walks me out of the stall.

"Has he been running in that unforgiving paddock? If so, his coffin bone is badly damaged. I specifically told you, Darlene, that Areion needs to walk and run on soft turf. He will not be able to stand all night. We need to put down more straw."

I try to stretch my neck down to reach the straw, but the pain in my left foot is unendurable and my level of discomfort is beyond anything I have experienced.

"I will have to call Dr. Alsace," my knight declares, casting a perturbed glance at Darlene, who remains silent.

"What? Dr. Alsace does not service this barn? Darlene, why didn't you mention this fact to me?"

Silence reigns, as Darlene realizes that no answer will be appropriate.

"A diagnosis cannot be given over the phone? But . . ." Roland's anxiety reaches a crescendo.

"I will give you my vet Tiffany's number. She is very competent," Darlene's tentative voice rings out.

Soon, I hear my knight say that Dr. Tiffany can only come on Friday afternoon. I have not the slightest idea when that time will come and I cannot say, in earnest, that it matters. For me, the only knowledge I have in this moment of eternity is pain. I am Areion, the Invincible! I chant in my soul, as Roland gives me bute[24] and curls up beside me. Sleep becomes our only escape, where we revel in the magic of the subconscious mind, where dreams of the heart become reality.

---

[24] Bute can be used as an analgesic for pain relief in horses.

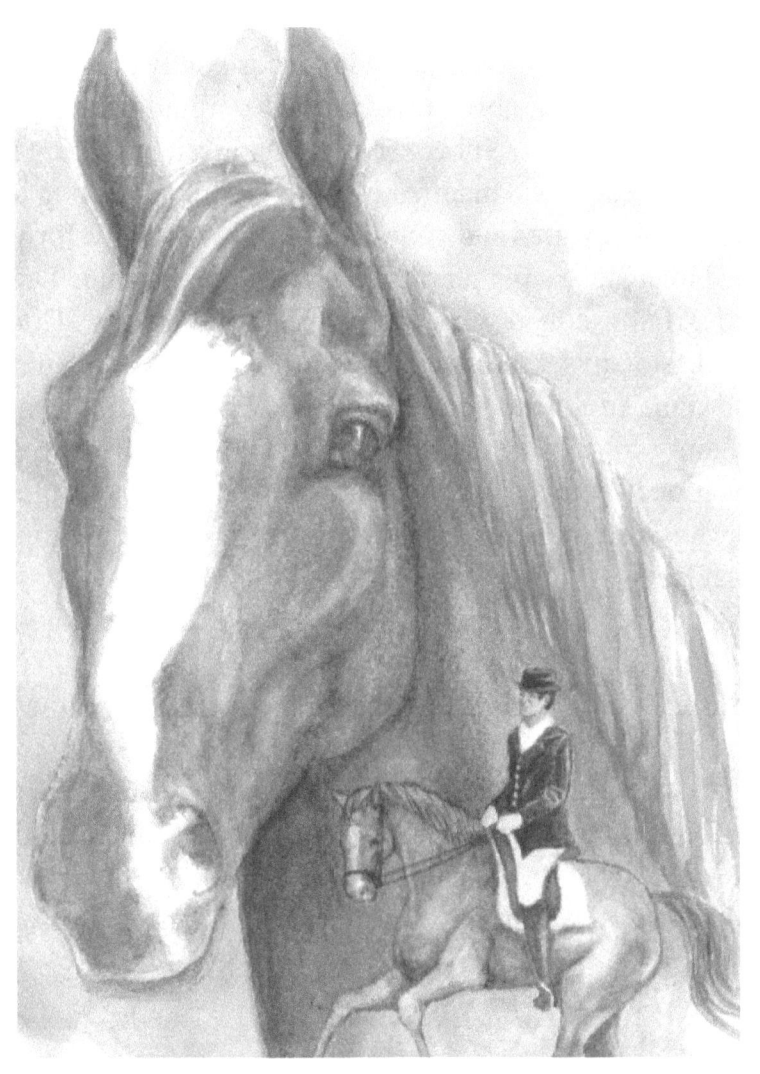

Chapter 14

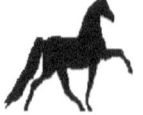

A Synchronized Reverie

wo brothers of one heart, with heads gently pressed in deep slumber, speak not! Quiet your weary minds, and allow me, your Collective Subconscious, Omniscient Receptacle of Dreams, to emerge and manifest your desire. Do not cling to life's daily residual thoughts and your painful waking reality, for you are destined to achieve a higher purpose in the dream-state. Dr. Freud himself acknowledged my governance in the matter. Confer to me permission to set the stage for your fondest wish fulfillment.[25] Roland and Areion nod in unison, and Subconscious assumes dominion.

All at once, Roland and Areion find themselves at High Brass Farm, whose trees display spring verdure. The two stop to imbibe the clean air.

"We are here again, my friend!" Roland exclaims, as he pats Areion's head.

Before Areion can react, the scene switches to the rehab center.

"Walk, Areion!" Mike Mebler commands, with gentle firmness.

Areion walks down the long aisle, approaches the treadmill, and enters lithely, as Mike elevates the water level.

"Mike, we're back! Can you believe it?" Roland appears, almost sprinting.

---

[25] In the following fictitious dream-sequence, "Subconscious," who becomes the objective, all-knowing narrator of Chapter 14, refers to Sigmund's Freud's theory that dreams are the expression of wish-fulfillments, the residue of latent daily thoughts (see Sigmund Freud's *Introductory Lectures on Psychoanalysis*, W.W. Norton & Company, Inc., London-New York, 1966, 226).

"Yes, and this great guy is doing better than ever!" Mike beams at Areion.

"I have no idea how this happened!" Roland looks about, with slight confusion.

"You have no time to think, Roland. The beginner's freestyle dressage show begins in just over a month, and you need a trainer.

"But, Mike, you don't allow outside trainers and, besides, Kati Regan is working in Florida now."

At the mention of Kati's name, Areion's ears perk up and he bellows like an elephant, wishing to say: "Tell my Kati to come anyway. We need her!"

"I will make an exception, this time, but it's our secret," Mike says good-naturedly. Set into motion, Roland quickly takes out his cell phone and speaks to Kati, whose sweet voice resonates throughout the center. Areion listens and tries to keep calm.

"Kati, Areion has improved greatly, and we need to begin our training as soon as possible. We have lost a lot of time but, now, things have turned around, and we have a chance to train for the beginner's show," Roland explains.

"Roland, I'm so happy for you, but I can't come right now. I have so many commitments and my employer, Barbara, needs me here. I hope that you understand. Please keep me posted."

Roland sulks, as he hangs up. Areion's ears sag and he ceases his workout.

"What are you doing, boy?" Mike looks puzzled. "You can't give up now."

Areion raises his head, stretches his neck, and looks in Roland's direction, as if to declare: "Me, give up? Never!" Acknowledging his cue, Roland approaches Mike.

"Since we don't have a trainer, Areion and I will work together independently in the indoor arena, where the ground is soft."

"Go for it!" Mike declares, raising a victorious fist in the air.

As Roland shakes Mike's hand, the scene transitions to an open field, where Areion stands in clover, neighing, in recognition of the harbinger of good fortune. Then, suddenly, the brothers appear in the indoor arena, where soft sand and dust invites them to commence training sessions. Recalling Kati's instructions, they accomplish basic movements, harmonizing physically and psychically in their mutual intention.

Though they work well together, they cannot fine-tune their practice and, ultimately, become frustrated. However, the two, ever reaching for the stars, never yield to despair, and experience some successful intervals of practice-time. Both feel free, entirely comfortable within their physical structures, not once remembering—or believing—that sorrow or pain ever have beset them.

On one particular occasion, after a good session, Roland begins to dismount, when he hears a familiar, melodious voice.

"Let's get started! Feet beneath you!" Roland turns to face a strong, athletic woman. He cannot believe his eyes and exclaims:

"Kati, what are you doing here? How did you manage to come back to New Jersey?"

"Hello, Mr. Areion!" Kati walks over to the appendix, who looks at her, nickering as though an angel has just appeared.

"My horse, Jake, has a suspensory ligament injury and has to be on stall rest for awhile. My boss, Barbara, is abroad in Germany, attending clinics, visiting friends and former trainers. So, I began thinking about how much freestyle dressage training means to you and Areion, and I will stay with you for six weeks, to help and guide you."

At that moment, Areion looks to the sky, as if to say: "Thank you, Universe, for bringing back my Kati!"

The scene switches to an overflowing field of grass and clover, where Areion romps and neighs, with abandon.

"Come out of there, Mr. Areion!" Kati commands, laughing.

"Dreams are good, but you have to work for them!"

With Kati as their mentor, Roland and Areion flourish, as they strive to harmonize their movements—psychologically and physically. In dressage, "harmony" connotes perfect balance, purpose and athletic expression in horse and rider. Roland begins to work on basic balance drills as he sits atop Areion.

"Harmony must come from your seat, your aids, and the absence of force," Kati instructs.

"That's it, Roland! Dominique calls out encouragingly, as she watches one afternoon. When Dominique is in attendance, the brothers are in their best form. Roland focuses on relaxed unison, rhythm and contact between his hand and Areion's mouth. The latter exercise enables control over and communication with the horse. Areion's dignified stance becomes more pronounced than ever, as he actualizes his lifelong dream.

"The wind once told me that my knight would come and here he is, here we are, an unbeatable team." Areion neighs excitedly.

"Shhhhhhhhhhhh!" Kati cautions. "Areion, you are disrupting the lesson. Your evenness, suppleness, obedience, and fluidity of motion are crucial. Your movements must be effortless. Kati's glances seriously at Roland. "Concentrate!"

Kati sees Roland's mind drift, as the scene transitions briefly and Roland goes back to Washington Stables, where he first took Western riding lessons. He looks frantically for Areion.

"Where is he, Connie? I can't find Areion! Is he gone?"

"Where is who? Who is Areion?" Connie inquires, materializing out of nowhere.

"Have I ever been without him? I must find my brother!"

The scene switches back to High Brass Farm. "Roland! Kati raises a concerned voice. Are you ill? If you don't focus, you will never get to the beginner's show! We're working on collection! You must practice 'Schwung,'" Kati continues, looking straight into her student's eyes. Watch me!"

"I'm with you, Kati." Roland returns to himself, thankful that he and Areion have not parted.

Kati explains the aforementioned term, "Schwung," to have derived from the German, "swing." In dressage, the word means movement and "swing" over the horse's hind legs, and is essential in collection. The latter engagement, in which all the necessary dressage elements combine, involves the lowering and increased prominence of the hind quarters, which allow the horse to come forward under the rider's weight.

"Ride on the bit, Roland. That's right. Drive Areion from behind and forward into soft contact with your hands. Very good!" Kati applauds her pupils.

The scene alters suddenly, and Areion's mind is with Flannery, the beautiful white ivory horse with a mutual inclination for knocking down fences.

"Come on, Flannery, my friend! Let's go!" he neighs, as the two miscreants charge into a fence.

"What is going on here?" someone calls out angrily.

"Uh, oh! We did it again! I'm in trouble with my knight!" Areion lowers his head.

The scene transitions back to High Brass, with Kati calling:

"Now, Mr. Areion, don't day-dream." We are almost done for today, and I can't have you wandering off."

Areion raises his head with customary pride.

"There you are!" Now, let's work on the gaits: the free, extended, and collected walks. You're doing very well. OK, now, the trots: walking, posting, extended and collected. Good! Now the canters, let's do them all, guys! Next, the half-halts, full-halts, and half-passes. Nice lateral movement! Excellent!" Kati coaxes. "Now, let's try twenty-meter circles in the corners of the arena," Kati makes a circular motion with her hand.

Areion looks at her as if to say: "I need a break. Can we stop for now?"

As if reading his mind, Kati offers a reply: "don't even think about resting, Mr. Areion. If you want to live your dream, you have to give everything within you. The twenty-meter circles are crucial for the musical kur routine."

"Do you think Areion knows anything about music, Kati?" Roland interjects, playfully.

"He knows about everything. His mind is as sharp as a tack." Kati recognizes Areion's keen senses and desire to perform with his rider.

The brothers and their adroit instructor continue to work on various movements: the half-volt, half-pass, zigzag at the trot, the serpentine ("snake-like" movement) at the walk and, then, at the trot, diagonal extensions, and, even flying changes, where Areion appears to skip across the arena at a canter. As Areion does this, marshmallow clouds seem to drift by. Areion neighs, as if to suggest: "We are touching the sky, Brother!"

Kati then challenges Areion to perform passage, wherein he appears to float, springing from one diagonal to another, while maintaining his body in a straight line. The brothers perform with such awareness and precision, that Kati is moved to tears. Not wishing to deflect from her pupils' purpose, however, she manages to maintain professional composure.

Time for the show grows near, and, with the proper support system, trainer, diet, left foot soaks, and an occasional treat, the brothers proceed on their way to becoming the true champions that they have always been—just as destiny intended.

"We will show everyone!" Roland is supremely confident, poised.

Time elapses before the team sets the elements to music, choreographed using the strength and agility of gymnastics, combined with the beauty and elegance of ballet. Roland chooses a piece which artistically conforms to the routine's aestheticism and serves, equally, as a personal metaphor: "He Ain't Heavy, He's My Brother,"[26] apropos of the indelible bond between horse

---

[26] One of the most enduring classics of the early 1960's, "He Ain't Heavy, He's my Brother was made popular by the English group, The Hollies.

and rider—most especially of two who have traveled a long road together, the horse unburdened by his rider's weight, bound by love, which makes all things possible.

Eternal time marches on in the mind's realm. Before the show date, Roland and Areion travel through the Province of Subconscious to visit Nacho in his new barn, happy to find that he has let go of the trauma of his past and is in very good form. A sojourn to the Silver Saddle's trailer horse area reveals that all of Roland's improvements have conduced to a better life for the horses. Without conscious acknowledgment of the changes around them, Betty and Dave's treatment of and empathy for their equine boarders has increased dramatically.

"Just one life can make a difference," Roland points out to his equine brother.

"And two can change the world." Areion neighs. In that instant, the brothers' hearts synchronize completely, and they stand poised and ready for their ultimate wish fulfillment.

The scene transitions to the U.S. Equestrian Facility in Gladstone, New Jersey. The brothers prepare by arriving one day early to acclimate Areion to the new atmosphere. Roland observes that Areion almost glides, free of any discomfort.

"Our miracle has happened, Kati!" Roland remarks to the tireless trainer.

"I always realized that Mr. Areion has the heart of a true champion," Kati replies tenderly. "I am proud of both of you!"

On show day, Kati and Roland equip Areion with his saddle, leaving his mane and tail flowing softly, his halter, and, finally, his full black leather bridal, engraved with his show name "Shadow's Pride." As never before, Areion stands erect, with his eyes focused on the horizon, consuming every moment of life, inhaling every ounce of air. His clean, white socks and bright copper-colored coat shimmer in the sunlight. Roland saddles him up, all the while rendering encouragement: "It took us a long time to get here, Brother. This is our moment. It is anyone's guess where life will lead us after this time ends, but that doesn't matter to me. What counts is this very instant and, no matter what happens at the close of this day, we have each other. Our strength is grounded in love, not in the judgment or approbation of others, not here or in any circle. Thank you for uplifting me, for taking me on this journey. Not once have you ever complained, but only have sought to love and be loved. Your courage has inspired and kept me on course. Very few have the opportunity to experience our type of connection. Many would have given up, but that notion was—and is—unthinkable to us. We share the difficulties, we celebrate the glory." Areion looks about at the beautiful, skilled horses around him, from black stallions to European warmbloods, bred to win. He nods in their direction, as if laden with doubt, saying:

"But, my knight, look at all of the others in our class! I feel like a misfit among nature's couture designs."

Roland smiles, as though he reads Areion's mind.

"Yes, you are different from these horses, my friend, but you must remember that, with your depth of heart, courage and desire, you cannot lose. You have a right to take your place with everyone. Stand your ground, keep your head high. We must believe in each other and work as one."

The scene alters again, as the brothers enter the warm-up arena. Scores of trainers, managers, sponsors, family and friends chant words of support, as they watch the magnificent horses walk, trot, canter, and perform some of their movements and transitions. Areion seems undaunted by the presence of the other horses, as he realizes that he has taken his place amongst those destined for career greatness. As he sports his trademark inner dignity and strength, he is transformed by supreme grace and beauty. Roland's demeanor also radiates with preparedness, as he faces the throng in dashing attire from head to toe. He wears a black derby, glistening riding boots of the same color, white gloves, riding pants and a jacket with tails. In the stands, Dominique (who has already rode and won her class with her mount, Princess Charming), her mother, Gerry, her father, Steve, and Kati look on, the latter calling out instructions:

"Sit back! Shoulders back! Loosen the reins and keep Areion relaxed! Keep the heels down and look up! That's right! Don't overdo! Just fifteen to twenty minutes of practice. We don't want Areion to breakdown or feel sore at the last minute."

The scene transitions to Kati beckoning Roland to move to the deck arena and, then, to the main show arena, where he awaits his turn. Roland looks to Areion for strength and courage.

My knight's heart is pounding in anticipation, Areion says silently, within. Please don't worry, my knight, we shall prevail, he says, in the spirit.

The crowd standing at the gates proceeds to the deck arena. Cheers rise up for the last contestant finishing a routine. Kati then declares, "You're next." Roland pulls himself together and pats Areion.

"This is it, Brother, our time in the sun. Risk, my friend, risk even failure, for you always were and will be my champion, my strength! We are one now!" Roland whispers, as Areion assumes a stance more regal than ever before. Roland begins to trot around the arena, as he hears a call over the loudspeaker: "Roland Stanzione and Shadow's Pride, up next! Their song is 'He Ain't Heavy, He's My Brother!'" A horn sounds and the music begins, as Roland walks down the centerline, stopping to bow to the judges. He drops his right hand and inclines his head, as Areion stands with eyes focused straight ahead, looking at a brilliant rainbow, visible only to the brothers, who believe in and manifest its existence. The two continue down the centerline, then left, and across the arena on trot, in time to the music. No sign of anxiety can be detected, even by Kati, the most observant of spectators. The twenty-meter circle seems easy for the pair, who stop at nothing to please, to give of their hearts, their greatest resource. They then proceed diagonally, reverse their path, turn right, go down the long side of the arena in a working trot, and turn right again. The lyrics "[. . . but] I am strong, strong enough to carry him" resonate poignantly, as Roland ponders: If Areion is in any pain, he still rises to this occasion, for he knows what the words mean.

Next, the team performs the half-pass to the left, turns, and proceeds in a twenty-meter circle, as the music reaches a crescendo. Shadow's Pride plunges deep within his spirit, as he keeps an eye on the rainbow, competing as if he were at Devon,[27] going from a canter to a trot, then transitioning into a flying change diagonally across the arena. "We're running with the wind together, my knight!" Areion's soul speaks aloud to Roland, audible to him alone.

"I realize that! Good boy! Now, focus! Transition to a trot down the long side of the arena. We're doing great!" Roland murmurs affirmatively.

Next, the brothers turn, begin a serpentine and, finally, turn left and execute a passage, a collected trot in slow motion, surpassing their level. Roland feels Areion float, maintaining balance and poise. Although applause are restrained during the performance, the audience cannot refrain from commending such a move at the lower level. Areion's confidence reaches its zenith, as he comes down the centerline and Roland triumphantly salutes the judges. At Gerry's, Steve's and Dominique's initiation, thunderous applause usher from the stands, as tears flow from Roland's eyes.

"Areion, look at that rainbow! Never have I seen so many colors!" Roland whispers. The two stand in statuesque posture, gazing outward. "This is all for you, Areion!" Roland adds, lovingly.

Since their performance occurred next to last, they wait a short time before the judges come back with results.

"Roland Stanzione and Shadow's Pride take the Blue Ribbon," an announcer declares over the loudspeaker. In the winner's circle, Roland dispenses with protocol and stays with Areion in the show arena. As if he and Areion are in the winner's circle having just won a stakes race, Roland quickly dismounts like a jockey, and falls to his knees, holding his head in his hands. He rises and hugs Areion,

---

[27] Thriving since1896, the horse competition at Devon, PA is the oldest, largest multi-breed event in the United States.

raising his fist to the crowd. "This is why we are here, Brother, not for the tangible award of the Blue Ribbon, but for this moment of victory, having conquered the odds!" He places the ribbon on Areion's halter, alongside his engraved name. "It is an honor to give this to you, my true friend! You did it, boy! You took a risk, treading on a road seldom traveled, with unparalleled heart and courage. You should be proud!"

At that moment, the brothers catch a fleeting glimpse of an unfamiliar face in the throng of on-lookers, that of a girl, smiling, with a single tear streaming down her cheek. She carries a sign which reads, "Areion Lives! Your story will be told!" As the brothers revel in lingering cheers, the girl vanishes into the multitude. The curtain of nighttime slowly unveils an impending dawn. Gradually, amidst the applause, Subconscious fades, along with the rainbow of many splendid colors.

Chapter 15

At Rainbow's End
(Roland's Narrative)

I cannot remember when I left Areion last night. I must have fallen asleep beside him and, then, returned home, at some point. I am consumed with worry, and my mind is in a fog. Nonetheless, I experience an odd sense of triumph, so incongruous with present circumstances. Oh, yes, now the reason is coming to me! I dreamed that my hero and I defied conventional definitions of "success" and "championship," that we received the Blue Ribbon in a beginner's dressage show. However, the prize did not elevate us (we were—and are—the same with or without such tangible acknowledgment); rather, the joy of proving ourselves before an audience of our peers, before skeptics, critics and naysayers, of living in the moment together, provided every ounce of our hearts' fulfillment. The dream seemed so real! I stop to ponder whether my subconscious theatrics actually occurred. I felt so free, and my Areion flew with the wind, and . . . where is the rainbow? I must be hallucinating. I must get to Areion—quickly. I just know that he ran on a hard surface which, no doubt, has caused potentially irremediable damage. There is nothing more to do other than run to his side.

A brief glance at the clock reveals the time to be 7:00 a.m. I rush to Areion's stall, and find him nibbling on some grain, in slightly better spirits. Should I expect anything else of my true champion, an exemplar of comebacks? I think to myself. Darlene informs me that Dr. Tiffany Marr will come at some time in the late afternoon. Areion and I spend the day together, awaiting the doctor's arrival. I take my beleaguered friend outside of his stall and over a driveway, as I observe his limp, today not as pronounced, but his foot still hurts on the hard surface. We walk to a big, open field, where the ground is exceptionally soft and moist after rainfalls. By now, fall has descended and the grass is fraught with dew and good for grazing. Areion gazes up at some of the other horses around him, neighing contentedly. As always, he does not allow his pain to disrupt the beauty of moments.

A noise in the driveway beckons our attention, and we look up to see the vet and Erica, her technical assistant, enter. Areion and I make our way back to the barn area to greet both. Dr. Tiffany is a pleasant, attractive, intelligent woman, eager to know about Areion's past. My equine friend senses, somehow, that our conversation centers on him. His intuitive abilities and appreciation of life always allow him to partake in human interaction.

I spend half an hour summarizing Areion's and my past few years together, explaining our dream of entering a beginner's dressage competition. Strangely, I feel as if the event already has occurred. I pause briefly to reflect on my dream, a fantastic, though misty, mental construct. Returning to myself, I observe Dr. Tiffany listening attentively, while posing a series of questions. She clearly empathizes with our situation.

"I understand your frustration, and admire your tenacity and devotion to Areion," she says, looking at me kindly. "Erica, trot Areion in a straight line. Let's see what's going on here," she instructs her young assistant. Areion trots off gingerly, revealing a pronounced limp in his left foot. Erica trots him twice more, with the same result.

"I am not optimistic, Roland." Dr. Tiffany addresses me morosely. "A beginner's show seems very much out of reach," she continues.

I wander briefly in thought, as I reel with sorrow. The dream had been an illusion, after all, a product of my desperate wish to save Areion's life.

Dr. Tiffany explains my hero's plight: "If Areion were to train for a show, conditions would have to be almost ideal. He would require a proper support system, training, rest, and great footing;

and, even under those circumstances, we have no guarantee that his foot would stand the test."

"If there is any way to beat the odds, Areion will find it," I affirm, reaching for a scintilla of hope. "He has such heart and strength of character. I just want him to be well, which is more important to me than anything."

"Would you agree to immediate digital x-rays?" Dr. Tiffany asks.

"Absolutely!" I reply, impatient for answers.

We take Areion inside, where Dr. Tiffany slightly sedates him and begins to take x-rays. All the while, I pat and rub my hero's head and neck. The all too familiar procedure and accompanying anxiety overwhelm me. Areion submits placidly, though I know, in my heart, that he is fighting to breathe freely, to be a horse, to run again. With everything in me, I wish this for him, for us.

Time edges in cruel increments as Dr. Tiffany looks at the x-rays. Her face clouds over.

"The news is not good," she says, decisively, with feeling.

I approach, as my pulse quickens. The x-ray-results look worse than those of Dr. Alsace.

"Areion's coffin joint is splintering," Dr. Tiffany explains. "The injury is analogous to having one's fingernail bent backward. The condition is called 'laminitis.'" My heart sinks and I become lightheaded. I manage, however, to reply, containing my overpowering grief.

"Areion is still young and wants so much to live. He ran on a hard surface, which exacerbated the condition. Can he undergo a surgical procedure to reverse it?"

"No, surgery and drug treatments will not serve now. The condition is far-gone. Areion cannot perform in this state." Dr. Tiffany places a gentle hand on my shoulder. "Can he just be a horse, then, grazing and running about?" I ask, nervously, awaiting some affirmation.

Dr. Tiffany speaks candidly. "The problem is that running will cause pain so severe that Areion will have to lie down."

If the rainbow has ever appeared, we have reached its end now, I think to myself. I repeatedly muse over everything I have done to keep Areion alive. The thought of competition is meaningless. The core issue is that my soulmate deserves far better than constant stall confinement and medical intervention. He has so much life within him, great love for me, and incredible zest for life. My miracle friend always has come through, my giver of strength. What can we anticipate now? I brood silently. Then, in an effort to avert the agony of my impending life-and-death decision, I force myself to be resolute.

"Do you think that I should put him down?" I ask, trying to appear stoic, while weeping in my heart.

"That is a big decision, which you must consider before proceeding," the doctor cautions.

"He is only thirteen, filled with life and energy. To restrain him from running and playing is unthinkable. He will not be himself, a horse who yearns to run with the wind, to be free," I answer, as my voice catches on every syllable. Then, after a few minutes' pause, I look to my hero and, then, at Dr. Tiffany. "I cannot dwell on the inevitable, and I cannot let him go through another night in such enormous pain. It's time . . . ."

"Are you sure that you don't want to think about this?" Tiffany and Darlene ask, in turn.

"Yes, I'm sure. In his condition, Areion faces a life of complete isolation. His spirit will be broken. My decision to end his suffering is my last gift to him, to allow him to roam freely in God's green pastures," I reply, as energy drains through my fingers.

Areion is alert now, listening to our dialogue, as I hold him on the lead line. He looks out at the barn grounds, peering to see whether the other horses remain outside. As Dr. Tiffany prepares the euthanization serum, Areion and I go to an outdoor arena for our last walk together. Dusk hangs heavily in the atmosphere. I pick up a blade of grass and show it to my hero. With tears streaming down my face, I can barely walk or speak, but I manage to address my friend.

"Do you see this, Areion? You took a simple blade and turned it into clover for me. You are life's most unselfish, pure and loving magician, having transformed my world into the most beautiful place. Never can I thank you for all that you have been to me. You will run with the wind again, Areion, and our paths will cross again, I promise! You were my strength, my guide in the present, my vision for the future. You saw my true self, rendering unconditional love, expecting nothing in return. Eternity will preserve our bond for all time, my friend and, while I live, so shall your memory, in my heart. I'm so sorry, so very sorry! I love you, best friend of mine!"

My tears flow endlessly, as I continuously utter the words: "I am so sorry! I love you!" Slowly, with tender reverence, I remove my hero's halter. Darkness takes hold as Areion gently kneels, a valiant innocent, yielding to the forces of life. As Dr. Tiffany inserts the first injection to put Areion to sleep, I sob uncontrollably into his neck, bending down in the arena's sand and stone dust

"Please hurry! I don't want him to linger or feel any pain!" I cry out.

Dr. Tiffany administers a second injection to stop Areion's heart. Suddenly, in a final display of unparalleled bravery and goodness, my friend opens his eyes and takes a last breath of farewell. At that moment, raindrops cascade around us, nature's manifestations of my immense grief.

Dr. Tiffany checks Areion's pulse, looks at me, and inclines her head. "I'm so sorry, she whispers."

With great kindness and empathy, Erica, the vet tech, offers me a long lock of Areion's tail and his left shoe, remnants of an essence whose loving heart exceeded the universe's expanse. To keep Areion's body warm, I cover him with the waterproof horse blanket I used whenever he played outside in light rain and snow.

My tears fall in torrents, into the night, as I kneel beside my hero. The sky hears my cries and offers a rainstorm of condolences. I am numb, unmindful of the elements, as I await the truck to come for Areion's cremation. I will keep his ashes, until my own life's curtain descends. Now, I am alone, as darkness encases me in desolation, without a rainbow in sight.

Chapter 16

I Am Spirit
(Areion's Message For Roland)

$\mathcal{M}$y knight, my brother, Roland, I am with you still, having slipped from earth's bounds in physical form alone. Now, I am spirit, truly immortal, racing with clouds and in beautiful fields of clover, pavements which your own love and tears have created. In letting me go, you unselfishly transcended the anguish and pain of loss and made ultimate sacrifice—all because you loved me.

In the face of rejection, you sought out and nurtured my inner qualities, at great sacrifice and risk, elevating me to heights of which I never dreamed. In and through you, I rejoiced in conferring and receiving love, the summation of life's supreme happiness. From you, I learned the art and grace of sharing, the harmony derived from friendship, and the strength of commitment. Such gifts surpass all championship ribbons. By your example, I learned that life is not, simply, a competition to win, but one of wills, in which the victor's true success comes from striving, respect for the game and all of its participants, irrespective of appearances. Grandeur inheres in the tiniest leaf, just as much as in the most elegant and fastest of thoroughbreds.

Nature does not discriminate but, when humans do, the underdog requires an advocate. You were my voice when society marginalized me and nearly dashed my every hope of life. Your name came to me on the wind, and I seized the opportunity of knowing you, my life itself. I found my purpose when I carried you, when we rode and dreamed together, as one.

Oh, yes, the dream! Never cease to believe that it existed—and does still! Someone special awaits you, a horse with a flowing black mane, whose name shall be Veillantif.[28] When you ride with him, look within, where you will find me, always giving you strength, cheering you forth, with the words: "My knight, keep your head up, with pride. I am not gone. I await you here, in my Creator's arms, until you come and we run together again, for all eternity. Now, cast away all shadows, dry your tears, and follow the pounding of my hoofs, running with the wind, as I gaze at the rainbow. Look, Brother! It's right before you!"

---

[28] The protagonist's horse in *The Song of Roland* (see Chapter 2 of this work).

Chapter 17

Commemoration

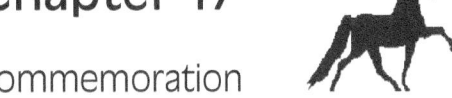

On October 27, 2007, the first anniversary of Areion's passing, I decide to pay homage by visiting the outdoor arena where he was euthanized. Bereft of my friend, I dwell in a moment of desolation. Sometimes, grieving is necessary to gain perspective, to mourn what has been lost, and to move forward. I don't attempt to stifle my tears, but pause to reflect on the one rose lying on the floor of my truck, which I intend to offer in tribute.

Clouds hang heavy in the sky and portend showers. How strange that history may repeat itself, I muse. As a steady light rain descends, the idea manifests. "Oh, Lord! I'm reliving last year all over again!" I utter aloud, but with full awareness that I am alone.

I drive up to the side of the barn, located on a rural, narrow road, and look out of my truck's passenger window. My gaze fixes on the spot where Areion died, as the rain grows steadier. I turn off my truck and bend down to pick up the rose, step out of the truck, and walk around to the side of the fence surrounding the outside arena. A late afternoon darkness comes over me. Areion, we are together, just like last year! I say silently, going deep within myself.

As the rain cascades around me, tears roll uncontrollably down my face. I begin to sense that Areion weeps with me, telling me that he misses and watches over me. I look at the rose in my hand, softly touch its petals, and then toss it over to the place where Areion drew his last breath.

Grief overwhelms me and I drop to my knees in the mud, invoking my friend's name. Hard times have beset me lately. I am out of work and don't know where my future lies. I always counted on Areion to nicker and listen to my joys and travails. Perhaps, somehow, he still can.

In the spring of that year, I edify a memorial in my backyard—lots of flowers, a small tree, a one-foot high picket fence, and a stone bearing his name—a befitting tribute to a remarkable life. His end was not finite, but only a beginning. My own heartbeat is evidence of this—the most telling vestige of a friendship that will surpass time.

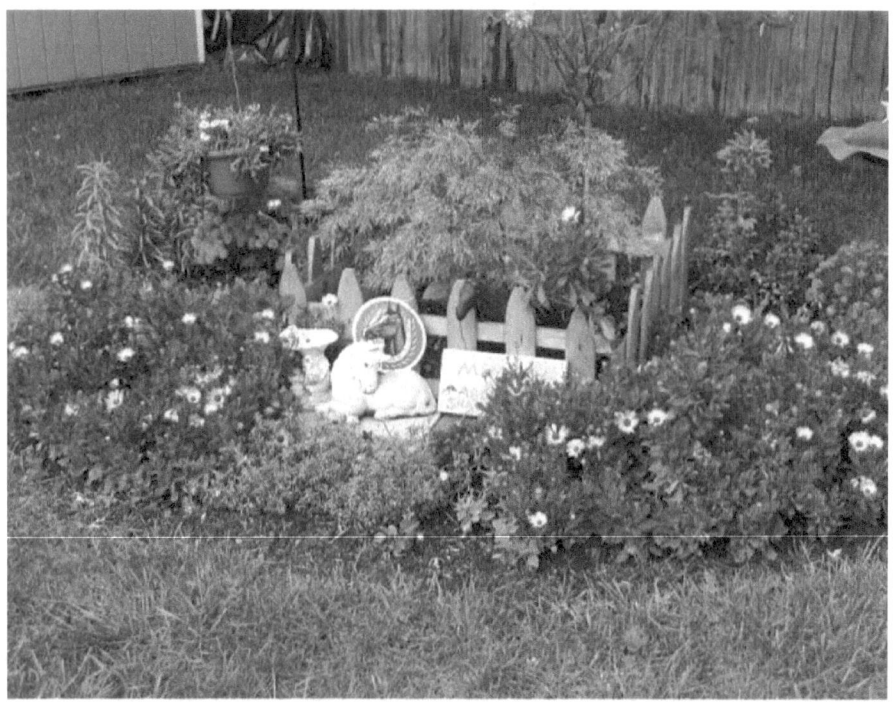

Chapter 18

Epilogue

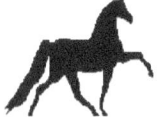

$\mathcal{M}$y friendship with Areion was one of the most pivotal, meaningful relationships of my life. Our connection raised my consciousness about life's challenges, in general, and about those on society's periphery, in particular, whether human or animal. The narrative, told from each of our perspectives, aimed to bring the reader into our combined and independent existences, in which we faced the vicissitudes of a highly unpredictable destiny.

Areion taught me to seize each day with a sense of wonderment, anticipation, and joy, despite all obstacles and misconceptions. Above all else, we wished to celebrate life and each other, irrespective of critical pronouncements from those in the "winner's circle." By this, I neither intend to glorify nor to denounce "winning," as the word is, customarily, defined but, rather, to point out that the term can have distinct meanings in a variety of circumstances. Every definition of "success"—and the life striving for it—has worth and merits a chance at fulfillment.

Areion knew that obstacles exist only in two places: in the mind's eye and in the hearts of those with tunnel vision. His ability to envision, never to give up, to grasp the moment, and to take pleasure in the smallest things (from a hug to a clover leaf, from breathing in the fresh air to running free of restraint) put my own life in context. In the process of trying to help my friend, I longed to raise awareness levels about him, to obliterate prejudicial roadblocks and negligence, which thwarted his chances of reaching his highest potential and, ultimately, of just being.

The cold reality of Areion's death demonstrated to me that, while attempts to change the collective consciousness may not always succeed, the immense joy and love given and derived from the effort makes the process supremely worthwhile. My hope is that Areion's legacy of determination, courage and love, as memorialized in these pages, has served to uplift and inspire those who, despite apparent failures or limitations, dare to live to their fullest capacity and to dream.